SECRETS *of* LONGEVITY

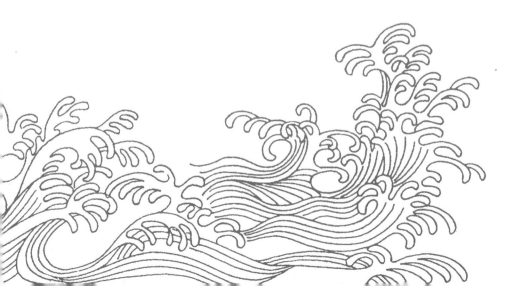

SECRETS *of* LONGEVITY

HUNDREDS OF WAYS
TO LIVE TO BE
100

by DR. MAOSHING NI

CHRONICLE BOOKS

SAN FRANCISCO

Library of Congress Cataloging-in-Publication Data available.

ISBN 10: 0-8118-4949-X

ISBN 13: 978-0-8118-4949-4

Manufactured in Canada

Designed by Laurie Dolphin Design

Design implementation by Folio2

Distributed in Canada by Raincoast Books

9050 Shaughnessy Street

Vancouver, British Columbia V6P 6E5

10 9 8 7 6

Chronicle Books LLC

85 Second Street

San Francisco, California 94105

www.chroniclebooks.com

Table of Contents

Introduction

Who among us doesn't want to live a long life? The desire to survive is built into us. As animals, we react instinctively to protect ourselves in the face of danger. As organisms, our bodies marshal natural defenses to fight off disease and heal injury. As social beings, we fondly hope to observe the new generations as they are born and grow. We all contemplate the seemingly mysterious differences among individuals—why do some people succumb to age-related syndromes while in their sixties and others live to be well over 100? We ponder the even more mysterious events imputed to "fate," when otherwise healthy people die from injuries or environmental affronts to the body.

I have had special reason to engage in such musings. An accidental fall from the rooftop of our three-story house when I was six years old left me in and out of a coma for a month and greatly weakened by the trauma. I am lucky that I was born into a medical family. My father was a doctor of Chinese medicine and a master of Taoist arts, and he and my mother rehabilitated me and guided me on the long road back to health. I still hold the memory of the herb teas' unpleasant taste, grueling early-morning tai chi and qigong practices, daily acupuncture sessions, meditation disciplines, and special food preparations.

The knowledge that made me whole again came from thousands of years of Chinese tradition of healing and rejuvenation, and I vowed that when I got well I would become a doctor and spread this tradition, to which I owed my life.

In 1985, while completing my postgraduate residency in Shanghai, I took note of the throngs of seniors converging at local parks every day at dawn to practice energy-enhancement exercises such as tai chi and qigong. I interviewed many of these seniors and even examined some of them. A good number were more than 100 years old. I was amazed at their grace and agility, sharp minds, vitality, and overall healthiness. This experience, combined with my recovery from that childhood accident, inspired me to explore a preventive approach to health, and thus began my twenty-year research effort on centenarians and the science of longevity.

The discoveries I made along the way fill this book. Marrying thousands of years of wisdom from the East with the latest scientific advances from the West, *Secrets of Longevity* provides time-tested and well-researched advice for achieving a long, healthy, and happy life.

To extend your life and improve its quality, you do not need to be in good health already. In other words, do not fret about the past. What you do from this moment on is what matters. The good news is that you can positively affect your health and longevity right now.

The causes of aging-related ills range from genetically pre-programmed cell death to destruction by environmental toxins to plaque and fibers that clog up the highways within our bodies. We all possess genes that are triggered as a result of how we live our life and the environment we are exposed to. Longevity is a matter of whether we express our good or bad genetic predisposition during our lifetime.

Unfortunately, Western society doesn't make it easy to increase our longevity potential. Our youth-driven culture and our neglect of the aged promote a wholesale denial of the realities of aging. The marketplace is full of products and devices promising to make us look and feel younger. In addition, conventional Western medicine focuses on treatment and replacement therapy, prescribing expensive drugs, removing a failed organ and transplanting a new one, or replenishing a depleted hormone. Very little emphasis has been placed on preventing disease and maintaining a vigorous state of health day to day.

In contrast, prevention and wellness have always been at the heart of Eastern medicine. Eastern doctors have long viewed disease as a symptom of life being out of balance. Therefore, the medicine they practice seeks to enhance and optimize health through diet, lifestyle, and emotional well-being. The Eastern paradigm also employs a variety of natural therapies such as acupuncture, herbal therapy, bodywork, tai chi, yoga, and meditation to treat the mind, body, and spirit. This approach empowers each individual in his or her pursuit of health and wellness.

Another important aspect of longevity is healing. At some point, due to factors beyond your control, you may become sick. How you handle the illness will have significant bearing on your longevity. Therefore, I recommend that you build a team of knowledgeable professionals dedicated to furthering your health and wellness. Seek out physicians who are willing to integrate complementary medical traditions such as acupuncture and herb remedies and who will take the time to educate you, answer your questions, and guide you in the pursuit of your longevity goals. As you read this book, become more aware of your health and seek treatment at the earliest opportunity— before a serious disease strikes.

The advice in this book is divided into five main chapters: What You Eat, How You Heal, Where You Are, What You Do, and Who You Are. By taking stock of these aspects of your life, you will be able to make changes needed to have increased energy, better memory, fewer colds, greater relaxation, more restful sleep, better sex, fewer ailments, and many other benefits. The final chapter, Bringing It All Together, synthesizes what you have read and encourages you to integrate the health techniques and life practices you have learned into a joyous, relaxed experience of being who you are. With discipline and a willingness to try the many tips in *Secrets of Longevity*, anyone who wants to live a long, healthy, and happy life has the ability to achieve it.

CHAPTER 1: What You Eat:
Diet and Nutrition

"I have heard that in the days of old, everyone lived one hundred years without showing the usual signs of aging. In our time, however, people age prematurely, living only fifty years. Is this due to our environment or is it because people have lost the Way?" asked the Yellow Emperor.

Qibo, his court physician, replied, "In the past, people practiced the Way. They understood the principle of the balance of yin and yang. Thus they formulated practices such as meditation to help maintain harmony with the universe. They ate balanced diets at regular times, arose and retired at regular hours, avoided overburdening their bodies and minds, and refrained from overindulgences of all kinds. They maintained well-being in body and mind, thus it is not surprising that they lived over one hundred years.

"These days, people have changed their ways. They drink wine like water, indulge in excessive eating and other destructive behavior, drain their essence, and deplete their energy. Seeking emotional excitement and momentary pleasures, people disregard the natural rhythm and order of the universe. They fail to regulate their lifestyle and diet, they sleep improperly. They do not know the secrets of conserving their energy and vitality. So it is not surprising that they look old at fifty and die soon after."

The Yellow Emperor's Classic of Medicine

This conversation between the Yellow Emperor, the first ruler of China, and his court physician took place some 4,700 years ago and is just as relevant today. As modern science has proven, the quality and quantity of the food you consume will have a lasting impact on longevity.

After examining the diets of approximately a hundred centenarians, I analyzed the data and correlated it with current anti-aging research. Not surprising, the diets and the studies dovetailed with the court physician's observations. The majority of centenarians lived by modest means, undereating was the norm among them, and some, due to circumstances more often than intent, practiced fasting for periods of time.

What the centenarians consumed, for the most part, was a variety of legumes, whole grains, vegetables, fruits, nuts, and seeds. Heavy carnivores were the exception—most ate a semivegetarian diet. These sound nutritional practices have been confirmed by Western science to contribute to health and longevity in a variety of ways.

In this chapter, you will find diet and nutrition tips ranging from foods with antioxidant properties to fasting practices for life extension. You are what you eat, so eat well.

     À votre santé! (To your health!)

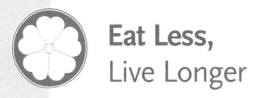

Eat Less,
Live Longer

After analyzing the diets of about a hundred centenarians, I found that the majority lived in modest circumstances. They ate less than the average amount, and some fasted at times because they were poor and simply had no food. Most centenarians surveyed around the world follow the "three-quarters" rule: they stop eating when they are three-quarters full. Studies have shown that a reduction in caloric intake can increase life expectancy in animals—why not humans?

Smaller Meals
More Frequently

Loading up our bodies with food three times a day is
a cultural habit, not a biological need. Instead, eating
smaller portions four to five times a day delivers a steady
stream of nutrients, blood sugar, and energy to the body
throughout the day. Less taxing on the digestive and
metabolic systems, smaller meals prevent overloading
and excess waste accumulation. Yet another benefit:
dividing caloric intake in this way reduces your risk of
heart disease.

Eat Like a King by Day,
Like a Pauper by Night

Remember the famous saying "You are what you eat"? It's also true that you are *when* you eat. Because of the human body's circadian rhythm, the same foods eaten at breakfast or lunch are processed differently than when they are eaten at dinner. Research shows that when you eat your daily protein and fat at breakfast you tend to lose weight and have more energy, while eating the same things at dinnertime produces tendencies toward weight gain, increased blood pressure, and heart disease.

Weekday Vegetarian,
Weekend Carnivore

Vegetarians generally suffer fewer degenerative diseases and cancers than their carnivore cousins. It's been estimated that a third of all cancer patients developed their disease as a result of insufficient whole plant fiber in their diets. However, you don't have to give up meat entirely to enjoy longevity—limiting your intake or eating meat only on weekends is a perfectly balanced and healthy approach.

Stay Alive:
Stop Eating Dead Foods

Ever wonder what Wonder Bread is really made of, or how many miles that head of limp lettuce has traveled? There's nothing like fresh, whole, organic foods to maintain your health and well-being. Farm-fresh produce and meats go directly from the source to your table, leaving little time in between for nutrients to be lost. Many foods at your supermarket have been picked or slaughtered weeks or even months before they make it onto the shelf. These items are preserved by nitrogen or other artificial means, making them appear fresh. Moreover, foods treated with pesticides and artificial fertilizers have lower nutritional value than foods grown organically.

Sweet Potatoes and Yams:
Not Just for Holidays

These powerhouse foods contain higher amounts of beta-carotene and vitamin C than carrots, more protein than wheat and rice, and more fiber than oat bran. Sweet potatoes and yams also happen to be a rich source of DHEA (dehydroepiandrosterone). This is a precursor hormone—a substance that remains latent until it converts into a hormone that the body needs. DHEA can become estrogen, progesterone, or testosterone, all essential for your body's anti-aging defenses to work. As one ages, however, the body's levels of precursor hormones like DHEA drop precipitously. Eat these vegetables year-round and celebrate a long life!

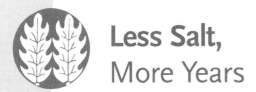

Less Salt,
More Years

Salt can preserve food, as sailors knew when they laid in their provisions for long ocean voyages. It doesn't preserve our health, though. Recent studies show that increased salt intake is proportional to an increase in cancers of the stomach, esophagus, and bladder. Additionally, sodium has long been implicated in chronic ailments such as heart disease, high blood pressure, and osteoporosis. Use other seasonings such as vinegar, garlic, herbs, and spices as tasty substitutes for salt.

Tea Party
Benefits All Guests

Celebrity testimonials are all well and good, but none of them can top this: tea is the beverage most commonly enjoyed by centenarians around the world. The free radical–inhibiting property of tea is more potent than that of vitamin E, and tea is a proven preventive and treatment for atherosclerosis (hardening of the arteries). The polyphenols in tea, especially the catechins, are powerful antioxidants that help ward off diabetes and cancer.

Ginger Gives
You Snap

Best known in the West for its antinausea properties, ginger has probably been in the longest continuous use of any botanical remedy in the world. The Chinese use it for both medicinal and culinary purposes, frequently in cooking seafood, since it acts as a detoxifier to prevent seafood poisoning. Besides its popular application for digestive distress, ginger has been found to contain geraniol, which may be a potent cancer fighter. It also possesses anti-inflammatory properties that help relieve pain, prevent blood clots, and inhibit the onset of migraine headaches. Since ancient times, Chinese physicians have regularly consumed ginger tea to keep their vitality fired up.

Little Wine,
Big Win

Extensive research has confirmed the benefits of wine
due to its high content of the antioxidant resveratrol.
This compound found in the skin of grapes possesses
anti-inflammatory properties and can reduce cholesterol
and prevent cancer. Wine also keeps the blood from
thickening in the blood vessels—preventing blood clots,
stroke, and plaque buildup. A little wine goes a long way,
however: only one glass a day is necessary to provide
benefits. If you drink more than a glass a day, the harm
may outweigh the good. So drink up—but just a little!

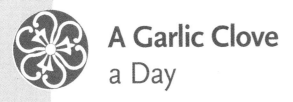

A Garlic Clove
a Day

The delicious ingredient that spices up Italian food does a lot more than whet your appetite. Studies indicate that allicin, the active ingredient in garlic, can prevent atherosclerosis and coronary blockage, lower cholesterol, reduce blood clot formation, stimulate the pituitary, regulate blood sugar, and prevent cancer. As an antibacterial, it is often used to treat minor infections. To balance out its pungency, eat some breath-freshening parsley.

Go Fish
for the Omega

If you're not a vegetarian, you'll want to make intelligent choices about the meat you eat. Of all animal products, fish is the healthiest, due to its high protein and low fat content. The omega-3 fatty acids in fish, along with other nutrients, protect blood vessels from plaque, reduce inflammation, prevent high blood pressure, and help you maintain good respiratory health. Populations with a diet consisting mainly of fish, fresh fruits, and local vegetables experience virtually no cardiovascular disease and have a high percentage of healthy seniors.

The Heart-
Happy Apple

The apple, a universally loved fruit, has long been a symbol of passion and temptation—and now, scientists have confirmed that it also contributes to a healthy heart. Eating two to three apples per day results in decreased cholesterol levels, thanks to the fruit's rich pectin content. Pectin also helps prevent colon cancer, which ranks among the top causes of death in adults over the age of sixty.

Brown Rice
for Long Life

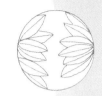

White rice begins as brown rice. Once the outer coating of rice bran is hulled off, however, not a lot of nutrients remain. A thousand years ago, Chinese physicians discovered that eating only refined white rice, devoid of the B vitamins in the bran, led to beriberi, a deficiency in thiamine (B_1). Modern research has identified a wealth of nutrients in the bran coating of brown rice. It is remarkably effective in lowering high blood sugar and therefore serves as an excellent food for diabetics. Rice bran contains more than seventy antioxidants, including the well-known aging fighters vitamin E, glutathione peroxidase (GPx), superoxide dismutase (SOD), coenzyme Q-10 (CoQ-10), proanthocyanidins, and inositol hexaphosphate (IP6). It is no wonder that rural farmers in Asia, who eat brown rice because white rice is too expensive, live longer and develop fewer health problems than their city-dwelling counterparts, who eat mostly white rice.

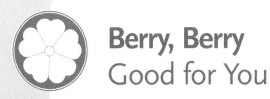

Berry, Berry
Good for You

Berries can be found in the wild in every region of the world. They are small fruits with intense flavors delicious to animals and humans alike. The dark red, blue, and purple skins of berries contain flavonoids that are more powerful antioxidants than vitamins C and E and more effective than aspirin at reducing inflammation. These anthocyanin flavonoids give cranberries their bacteria-fighting properties and may be responsible for lowering cholesterol as well. The blueberry, however, has been shown to have the highest level of antioxidant activity. Blueberries have neuroprotective properties that can delay the onset of aging and age-related memory loss by shielding brain cells from damage by chemicals, plaque, or trauma.

Eat Your
Sea Vegetables

Seaweed and marine algae are vegetables from the sea that have long been considered to possess powers to prolong life, prevent disease, and impart beauty and health. Common types of seaweed include nori (sushi wrap), kombu, kelp, dulce, and Irish moss. Containing more calcium than milk, more iron than beef, and more protein than eggs, seaweed is also a rich source of micronutrients. Traditionally, its healing properties are said to include shrinking goiters, dissolving tumors and cysts, detoxifying heavy metals, reducing water retention, and aiding in weight loss. So eat your sea vegetables! They have more concentrated nutrition than vegetables grown on land.

B's and C's Get
an A in Nutrition

When your mother told you to eat your broccoli, she was already looking out for your longevity. Cruciferous vegetables are potent defenders against cancer, the number one killer in industrialized societies. The crucifers are made up of the B's (broccoli, bok choy, and brussels sprouts) and the C's (cauliflower and cabbage). These vegetables contain phytonutrients that help cleanse the body of cancer-causing substances. One of these compounds, indole-3-carbinol, is a powerful antiestrogen that counters cancerous growth in the estrogen-sensitive cells found in the breasts, colon, and prostate. Crucifers are also a good source of beta-carotene, vitamins C and E, folate, and calcium, most of which are also antioxidants.

Sow Your Oats!

Oat bran, the outer coating of oats, contains high concentrations of soluble fibers, which help trap cholesterol and move it quickly through the intestines. Unfortunately, most people eat their oats in the refined form, which contains very little of the precious bran that contains beta-glucan and saponins. Whole oats are also rich in the antioxidants that stop cholesterol oxidation, the process that enables it to stick to artery walls.

More benefits: oats prevent colon cancer by binding toxic minerals and acids; they balance the body's blood sugar levels by slowing the absorption of carbohydrates; and the saponins in oats increase production of natural "killer cells," a critical part of the body's immune surveillance system. Try substituting a warm bowl of whole oats for your cold cereal in the morning. Your body will thank you— for years.

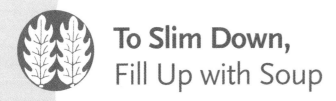

To Slim Down,
Fill Up with Soup

Obesity has become epidemic throughout the industrialized world. As a result, the rates of heart disease, stroke,
cancer, and diabetes are rising with alarming speed. One
simple dietary change can cut your risk of being counted
in the premature death statistics—eat soup at least once
a day. A nutritious soup that is low in salt rehydrates as it
nourishes and flushes waste from the body. Bottom line:
people who eat one or more bowls of soup each day lose
more weight than those who eat the same number of calories but don't eat soup. Homemade is best, as canned
soups are loaded with salt and chemicals.

Good Fat,
Bad Fat

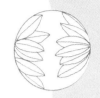

Not all fats are bad ones. Here's how to tell the helpers from the hurters. There are three types of fat: monounsaturated, polyunsaturated, and saturated.

Monounsaturated fats such as olive oil, sesame oil, canola oil, almond oil, flax oil, and fish oil are good fats. They contain essential fatty acids such as omega-3 and gamma-linolenic acid (GLA) that are critical in brain development and function, vascular health, proper immune function, skin health, fertility, and normal physical development.

Polyunsaturated fats—margarine, hydrogenated safflower oil, sunflower oil, and corn oil, among others—also contain essential fatty acids. However, these fats are highly refined and contain large amounts of trans fat (created when vegetable oils are hydrogenated to make them spreadable), which is implicated in heart disease and cancer.

The bad fats are the saturated fats and trans fats produced by deep frying: butter, palm kernel oil, peanut oil, coconut oil, and lard. These bad fats elevate cholesterol and triglyceride levels, increasing the chance of heart attack and stroke. Best to avoid them.

Chew It Up

To live longer, be kind to your insides. How? Each time you take a bite of food, chew at least thirty times before swallowing. When you do, your food is predigested in the mouth by the enzyme ptyalin, found in your saliva. As a result, the stomach doesn't have to work as hard, and absorption of important vitamins and nutrients occurs more readily. As I tell my patients, your stomach doesn't have teeth! It breaks down food with nothing more than gastric juice and acid. Eating too quickly also contributes to an increased production of acid, resulting in the common problem of heartburn, also known as gastroesophageal reflux disorder (GERD). Another benefit of chewing thoroughly is that you will feel full after eating less food, keeping your weight at a healthier level.

Don't Kill Your Food

To get the most out of the good things in your foods, treat them gently. High heat cooks away many important nutrients. Boiling, for instance, can destroy half of the vitamins found in vegetables. Deep-frying yields fatty foods and produces the worst kind of fat—trans fat—which can clog your arteries and increase your risk of cancer. Similarly, your cancer risk may rise if you make a habit of eating barbecued or grilled meat that is burnt or blackened. Try not to kill your food with too much fire. Instead, lightly steam, quickly stir-fry, or broil foods to preserve their nutritional value.

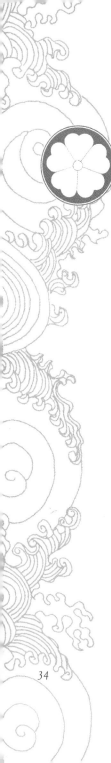

"Anti-Rust" Nutrients

Aging causes oxidation, which literally means rusting. As you get older, "rust" forms everywhere in your body in the form of waste buildup—uric acid from digesting protein, lactic acid from muscle use, carcinogens ingested or inhaled from the environment—resulting in creaky, painful joints and clogged arteries. Antioxidants are "antirust" nutrients that neutralize and remove the free radicals that cause oxidative damage. Among the many antioxidant nutrients, glutathione is considered the "master antioxidant." A naturally occurring compound found in asparagus, avocado, walnuts, and fish, it is composed of three amino acids: glycine, glutamic acid, and cysteine. Glutathione regulates immune cells, protects against cancer, aids DNA synthesis and repair, assists in detoxifying, and inhibits the activation of dormant HIV virus. A deficiency in glutathione can be a factor in diabetes, low sperm count, liver disease, heart disease, and premature aging.

Nuts and Seeds
Keep You Young

Just a handful of nuts and seeds every day can help improve
circulation and muscle tone. Arginine is an amino acid
found in soy and other beans, seafood, whole grains, eggs,
dairy, brewer's yeast, and especially abundantly in nuts and
seeds. It is a nonessential amino acid, a substance our bodies
produce in the liver and deplete during times of stress.
Arginine is helpful in fighting heart disease, impotence,
infertility, and high blood pressure as well as facilitating the
healing process. Its anti-aging properties may lie in its stim-
ulant effect on the pituitary gland at the base of the brain.
The pituitary releases growth hormone, which declines rapidly in humans after age thirty-five. Lower levels of growth
hormone contribute to symptoms of aging such as fat
deposits, decreased muscle mass and strength, cognitive
decline, and sexual dysfunction.

Password to a Treasure of Health: Open Sesame!

The most common oil consumed by Chinese centenarians, sesame oil is enjoyed for its refined, nutty flavor but possesses therapeutic properties as well. Chinese medicine lists sesame as a kidney and liver tonic, a blood builder, and a bowel protector and regulator. Sesame is rich in phytic acid, an antioxidant that may prevent cancer. The oil of one variety, lignan sesamin, was found to drastically reduce cholesterol levels in the liver and bloodstream of rats. To enhance flavors and improve health, sprinkle sesame seeds and oil in your food regularly.

Growth Hormone
from Eggs and Grains

Human growth hormone (hGH) has moved to the fore-front of anti-aging treatment, dramatically improving many elderly patients' lives. Primarily used to treat children with delayed growth, hGH also aids the frail by improving healing, tissue repair, brain function, bone strength, energy, and metabolism in general. Its benefits, however, come at a high price: a decided increase in the risk of cancer. Only if the patient's body no longer responds to natural stimulation—nutritional and herbal supplements, acupuncture, and energy-enhancement exercises—will I suggest such therapy. For the majority, I recommend boosting the natural production of hGH with GABA, or gamma aminobutyric acid. An excellent substitute for growth hormone, GABA is a nonessential amino acid found in soy and other beans, seafood, whole grains, eggs, brewer's yeast, nuts, and seeds. Especially after exercise, eating GABA-rich foods stimulates the pituitary to secrete hGH.

Vim
and Vinegar

In your quest for longevity, look to those who have found it. Apple cider vinegar has been a part of the health regimen of centenarians throughout the world. Its acetic and butyric acids promote gastrointestinal health by balancing pH and encouraging friendly bifido bacterial growth. Vinegar has antiseptic and antibiotic properties; it may also help to reverse atherosclerosis, or hardening of the arteries, and dissolve gall and kidney stones.

Honey,
the Natural Antibiotic

Long known for its antibiotic properties, honey is also
much more nutritious than refined table sugar, which lacks
the vitamins and minerals natural honey contains. Honey-
soaked gauze used to bandage burns and wounds can
also aid in healing. As a folk remedy, honey has been taken
for stomach ulcers and heartburn, and Western research
indicates that it may stop the growth of *H. pylori*, the bacteria responsible for most gastric ulcers. The caffeic acid
in honey may also prevent colon cancer. There's just one
caution with this delicious, nutritious, bacteria-fighting
sweetener: because raw honey can harbor botulism
spores, never give it to a child under one year of age.

The Ultimate
Longevity Food

In Asia, mushrooms are favored for both their taste and their therapeutic value. Chinese legend is filled with stories of those who discovered the 1,000-year-old mushroom and became immortal. An underground stalactite cave museum outside of Kunming, China, displays a reishi or ganoderma mushroom that measures 4 feet in diameter and is estimated to be about 800 years old! There are more than 100,000 varieties of mushrooms, about 700 of them edible. Many mushrooms, particularly shiitake, maitake, reishi, and wood ear, have superb anti-aging properties. Depending on the type, they may contain poly-saccharides, sterols, coumarin, vitamins, minerals, and amino acids that boost immune function, lower bad cholesterol, regulate blood sugar, and protect the body from virus and cancer. And you don't have to dig for them in the mountains any longer—they're readily available in your local health or specialty food store.

Be Healthy
as a Weed!

Burdock has long been known for its ability to thrive and propagate—witness its proliferation throughout the eastern part of the United States, where the plant spreads like wildfire along roads and hillsides. Recently categorized as an adaptogen (a natural substance that aids the body during stress and environmental changes), the root of burdock has been used as both food and medicine in Asia and Europe for thousands of years. Traditionally made into a nourishing tonic to speed recovery from illness, it has also become popular for functional support in rheumatism, liver disease, and cancer. Burdock root is a regular part of the diet among the Japanese, who have the longest life span in the world.

Secrets of
the Evergreen

In ancient times, Taoists living in the mountains of China observed that during snowy winters the only plants exhibiting vitality were evergreens such as pines. Through experimentation, they found a therapeutic use for every part of the pine tree: a physical and mental energy boost from pine needle tea and bark tea, antimicrobial properties in sap, and sustenance from pine nuts as a food. Since then, the pine has become a symbol of longevity in Chinese culture.

A potent antioxidant in pine called pycnogenol protects endothelial cells (which make up the lining of the blood vessels and heart) from free radical damage, serves as an anti-inflammatory, and preserves healthy skin structure. It is one of only a few antioxidants that cross the blood-brain barrier, protecting brain cells from the ravages of free radicals in the blood. Pycnogenol is available in dietary supplement form, but the same beneficial flavonoids can be obtained by eating pine nuts.

The Cancer-Fighting Tomato

Tomato's red pigment, called lycopene, is an antioxidant that has been studied extensively for its cancer prevention properties. Eaten in high quantities, tomatoes can lower the risk of prostate, stomach, colon, and rectal cancer. Lycopene also inhibits the development of cancer cells in the breasts, lungs, and uterus. A rich source of beta-carotene and vitamins A and C, tomatoes are also known to reduce heart disease and prevent cataracts. Not bad for a fruit regarded as deadly in some parts of the world as recently as the early 1800s. (A note of caution: people with arthritis and other autoimmune disease symptoms may be aggravated by eating tomatoes.)

Sea Salt
for Essential Minerals

Before we were born, we spent nine months in a bath of amniotic fluid resembling the primordial saltwater from which life arose. No wonder the human body contains fluids closely resembling the composition of the ocean. Sea salt contains nearly sixty trace minerals essential for the formation of vitamins, enzymes, and proteins that keep our bodies going. Salt aids in general detoxification, and its alkaline quality helps balance the overly acidic pH environments that breed degenerative and cancerous conditions.

Common table salt, however, is refined to nothing but sodium chloride and is devoid of all other essential minerals. I suggest using only unrefined sea salt such as that found in the salt beds of Brittany, which has a slightly gray hue. Of course, salt is to be used only in moderation, especially for those with hypertension. (See *Less Salt, More Years* on page 18.) It is also important to balance salt intake with potassium to ensure proper nerve and muscle function; potassium-rich foods include leafy vegetables, soy, whole grains, potatoes, bananas, and most fruits.

Liquid
Longevity

From time immemorial, water has been highly regarded for its therapeutic virtues. Centenarians on every inhabited continent swear by their native water as the source of their long lives. Scientists agree that these particular waters may contribute to the local inhabitants' health and longevity. One thing they all have in common is purity: no chemicals, no toxins. And it's no surprise that these Shangri-las are all located far from any city. Tap water in urban areas contains pesticides, industrial pollutants, chlorine, fluoride, and other chemicals. Well water and mountain streams in some parts of the countryside fare no better due to acid rain and toxic levels of minerals present in groundwater.

There are many filtration processes that remove contaminants. The best kinds employ activated charcoal, which removes the impurities but leaves the water-soluble minerals. Avoid water softeners, which remove essential minerals, and do not store water in plastic containers, as the polychlorinated biphenyls (PCBs) leach into the water.

An Anti-Inflammatory
on Your Salad

Native to North America and Asia, evening primrose has been used by American Indians and Asians alike for centuries to ease the ills of arthritis, stomach disorders, sore throat, hemorrhoids, and bruises. Evening primrose oil contains a rich supply of gamma-linolenic acid (GLA), an omega-6 fatty acid that aids in reducing inflammation; thus it helps combat rheumatoid arthritis, nerve damage, and Alzheimer's-induced memory loss. Because GLA aids the transmission of nerve impulses, it may also be helpful in multiple sclerosis. Evening primrose comes in capsule form or as an oil. Go ahead and use it in salad dressing!

Best Color for Healthy
Blood: Cherry Red

Chinese researchers have long observed that cherries help keep diabetics healthy. The antioxidant compounds that impart the dark pigments to cherries, grapes, and berries have been found to increase insulin production in the pancreatic cells of animals. Known as anthocyanins, the compounds also protect you against heart disease, cancer, and arthritis. So load up on cherries and other dark-colored fruits to maintain balanced blood sugar and enjoy a healthy old age.

Olive Oil Optimizes
Blood Pressure

Olive oil, long a staple of the Mediterranean diet, has been shown to have beneficial effects on blood lipids and may also lower blood pressure. About 60 percent of strokes and 50 percent of heart disease are attributable to high blood pressure, according to the World Health Organization. Hypertension is estimated to be responsible for 7.1 million deaths per annum worldwide. According to a recent study, "Olive oil intake is inversely associated with both systolic and diastolic blood pressure." Translation: consuming more olive oil is linked with lowered blood pressure. Use olive oil both for cooking and on salads—your blood pressure will thank you.

Carbonation:
Bad for Bones

Beverages with bubbles contain phosphoric acid, which is harmful to calcium metabolism and diminishes bone mass. This means that drinking sodas and carbonated water increases your risk of osteoporosis. Sometimes carbonation occurs naturally, as in certain spring water, but unfortunately this, too, has high levels of phosphoric acid. If you're going to live a good long time, you'll need healthy bones, so it's best to choose teas, light juice blends, and flat spring water to quench your thirst.

Be a
Decaf Detective

When you experience stress, anxiety, a racing mind, or insomnia, you already know what to do: cut out the caffeine. It's a central nervous system stimulator that works against your attempts to relax the body and calm the mind. If you still enjoy the taste of coffee, you might turn to the decaffeinated version—but beware. Many commercial coffees decaffeinate with methylene chloride, a chemical that interferes with the blood's ability to deliver oxygen. This causes the heart to work harder in an attempt to supply the needs of all the cells. If you have angina and have switched to decaf to avoid triggering symptoms, you'll want to be sure your brew has been swept clean of caffeine (well, 97 percent clean) using a water process. Check the label when buying coffee beans at your health food store, or ask the server at your café.

Orange Rind
Peels Away Cholesterol

In Chinese medicine, orange peel has been traditionally used to improve digestion of fatty and rich foods, and in Chinese cuisine it is often found in dishes with red meat. Orange peel may actually lower cholesterol better than some current medications, and without the side effects. Studies show that compounds called polymethosylated flavones (PMFs), found in pigments of oranges and tangerines, reduce bad cholesterol (LDL) without altering the level of good cholesterol (HDL). The next time you prepare a meal that's on the fatty side, make sure you use orange peel as one of the ingredients.

You Can Literally
Eat Your Heart Out

Overeating is one of the worst forms of stress on your heart. When you overeat, you tax every system of your body and increase the burden on your cardiovascular system. But most important, when the stomach distends from excessive food volume it compresses the aorta and the arteries around the upper abdomen and pushes up against the diaphragm. This restricts both lung and heart movement, potentially leading to serious heart disease. Be good-hearted and eat moderately.

Spice Up
Your Circulation

The natural reaction to eating spicy food is redness in the face, increased body temperature, and perspiration. These are signs that your blood vessels are dilated and blood flow is accelerated. Many spices, especially garlic, onions, cayenne, and turmeric, have been clinically shown to prevent blood clots and improve circulation. To help your blood keep you healthy, add spices and let it flow.

Housekeeping
for the Body

Plant fiber, called cellulose, acts like a broom to sweep the intestinal tract of toxins. It also inhibits the liver from producing cholesterol and draws out built-up bile, which can cause stones and jaundice. Three foods rich in cholesterol-busting fiber are oat bran, soy, and grapefruit. Choose your broom and sweep clean.

Packaged Food's
Unwelcome Additives

The three most common food additives used to preserve color, prevent spoilage, and enhance flavor in packaged foods are sulfites, nitrates, and MSG (monosodium glutamate). Sulfites can cause severe allergic reactions like asthma. Nitrates combine with amines in foods to form nitrosamines, which can lead to neurological damage or cancer. Headaches are commonly associated with MSG, and high levels of the substance induce blindness in animals. Other additives such as artificial colors and flavors also cause cancer in animals. To live long, avoid additives in foods—whenever possible, buy all natural.

You Eat Naturally—
Does Your Food?

Conventional meat, poultry, and dairy products contain high amounts of pesticides, hormones, and antibiotic drugs that are harmful to your health. Add the risk that your meat comes from diseased animals raised in stressful, inhumane conditions, and you have a good case for converting to vegetarianism. Commercial feed for animals is full of growth-stimulating hormones, coloring agents, pesticides, and drugs. And that's not all—of the 140,000 tons of poultry condemned annually as unfit to eat, mainly due to cancer, a considerable amount is processed into animal feed! More than 40 percent of antibiotics produced in the United States is used as animal-feed additives. The ecological result, after we urinate and defecate the antibiotics, is the emergence of antibiotic-resistant bacteria strains that can sicken or kill us. Whenever possible, buy only organic and free-range animals for your health, peace of mind, and well-being.

Broccoli
for Breathing

Our life expectancy is directly proportional to our lung capacity. For the majority of people living in or near metropolitan areas, traffic and secondhand smoke vastly accelerate loss of breathing capacity and increase the incidence of lung cancer. However, antioxidant-rich vegetables and fruits such as broccoli and apples can help mitigate these effects. One study revealed that subjects who ate more than five apples a week had better lung function than those who ate no apples. It's also been shown that the antioxidant isothiocyanates in cruciferous vegetables like broccoli substantially reduce lung cancer risk.

Bulk Up Bones
with Orange Juice

Bone loss, a slow, inevitable part of the aging process, can lead to life-threatening bone fractures if it becomes excessive or progresses too rapidly. Calcium and vitamin D are both crucial to bone health. Traditionally, cow's milk has been touted as the ideal food for strong bones, but many people react adversely to lactose. Now studies show that your body is capable of absorbing vitamin D and calcium from orange juice as readily as it does from milk. Besides being good for your bones, orange juice is also full of vitamin C, a potent antioxidant.

Spices Make the
Most of Your Food

Digestion takes many organs all working together to break down, absorb, and process the myriad nutrients in your food. Without healthy digestion, malnutrition may occur and toxins can build up in your body, causing rapid aging and degenerative diseases. Symptoms of poor digestion include bloating, gas, indigestion, constipation, diarrhea, and fatigue. Many common cooking herbs and spices are helpful in aiding proper digestion. These include dill, oregano, basil, coriander, rosemary, bay, ginger, fennel, anise, cardamom, and others. Use them in your cooking or steep them as tea to drink after meals.

Eat Your Spinach
for Better Eyesight

Popeye knew all along that spinach makes you strong, and now studies suggest that it also helps you see better. Each year, one in six Americans age fifty-five or older develops macular degeneration, and 1.2 million suffer severe vision loss. Spinach is full of the antioxidants lutein and zeaxan-thin, which protect the retina from age-related macular degeneration. And since fat increases lutein absorption, don't forget to sauté your spinach with a little olive oil.

Sorghum Beats Wheat— and Even Brown Rice!

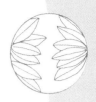

Here is an anti-aging food that most people in the West have not heard of: sorghum. Many Chinese centenarians eat sorghum as the main element in their diets, especially when rice is scarce during poor harvests. Sorghum, one of the first grains to be cultivated, is easy to grow and was a staple in China for millennia until rice replaced it as the main dietary grain. Ironically, sorghum contains more antioxidants, including vitamin E, than brown rice. Additionally, sorghum's bran layer has more insoluble fiber than wheat bran. Sorghum flour can be used as a substitute for wheat flour in baking.

Artichoke: First Aid for Your Liver

Due to the chemical assaults of the world we live in, most people's livers are overburdened by chemical overload and function sluggishly. Artichoke to the rescue! This delicious vegetable is also a potent liver protector due to a flavonoid called silymarin. Silymarin has strong antioxidant properties, and studies on animals indicate that it may protect against liver toxicity and cancer. So next time it's in season, steam and eat a couple of artichoke flowers to keep your liver humming along.

Cancer and Fat:
The Stats

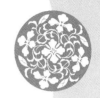

People in the United States consume an enormous amount of fat in their diet, often 40 to 50 percent of their total daily calories. High-fat animal-derived foods have repeatedly been correlated with cancer: studies show that men and women who eat meat every day, or consume butter or cheese products three or more times a week, are three times as likely to develop breast cancer and prostate cancer as those who eat these high-fat animal foods seldom or not at all. Your body needs fat, so treat it to the good kinds. These include fats and oils from legumes, beans, and other vegetables as well as nut and seed sources.

When It Comes to Protein, Less Is More

The Western obsession with protein diets is turning out to have potentially fatal results: osteoporosis and kidney failure. During protein metabolism, your kidneys must excrete the excess components of protein, namely amino acids. To complete this process, the kidneys neutralize the acids by binding them to calcium, depleting your body's store of this essential mineral. The U.S. rate of osteoporosis is dramatically higher than that of China, where the majority of people eat a lower-protein vegetarian diet. There's also evidence that excess protein weakens kidney function. In studies of animals with chronic kidney failure, simply reducing protein intake extended their life span by up to 50 percent.

Eat Low
on the Food Chain

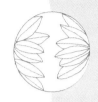

Since the Industrial Revolution, man-made chemicals and toxins such as pesticides, herbicides, heavy metals, and radioactivity have been polluting our environment and finding their way into our food supply. The higher you go on the food chain, the more concentrated these toxins become and the greater the danger they present. For example, in the ocean the creatures at the top of the food chain are large fish such as swordfish and tuna, which eat smaller fish that eat even smaller fish, and so on. At the end of the chain, the tiniest fish eat plants such as algae and botanical plankton. The toxins in each fish's body become condensed in this process, and thus the large fish contain the highest levels of these poisons. For land animals like ourselves, the best idea is to eat at the very bottom of the food chain: beans, legumes, fruits, nuts, seeds, and other plants, making sure they're organic.

Don't Be
Foiled by Oil

Oils from vegetable, nut, and seed sources provide us with essential fatty acids that are critical for nerve and brain functions. Typical vegetable oils bought at supermarkets, however, are not only potentially filled with pesticides but have been subjected to chemical and heat processing that reverses their value—extraction, distillation, cooking, refining, bleaching, defoaming, and the addition of preservatives—as well as exposure to light and air. All of this destroys the quality of the oil and causes the formation of free radicals, which completely defeats the purpose of consuming essential fatty acids. Buy organic, cold-pressed, minimally processed oils at your local health food store, and make sure that you consume it within three months. Olive oil, walnut oil, flaxseed oil, and soy oil are excellent choices. Store your oil in the refrigerator in dark glass containers to prevent rancidity.

Sugar's Side Effects
Aren't So Sweet

The average American consumes nearly 240 pounds of sugar per year. Most of the excess sugar is stored as fat in your body, which elevates cancer risk and can suppress your immune function. When study subjects were given sugar, their white blood cell count decreased significantly for several hours afterwards. This held true for a variety of types of sugar, including fructose, glucose, honey, and orange juice. In another study, rats fed a high-sugar diet had a substantially elevated rate of breast cancer compared to rats on a normal diet. To live long, draw sweetness from other aspects of your life.

The Bitter Truth About
Artificial Sweeteners

It's amazing to me how many health-conscious individuals will not think twice about drinking a diet soda that's filled with artificial sweeteners such as aspartame, sucralose, or saccharin. All of these artificial sweeteners pose dangers to one's health and longevity—saccharin, for example, has been found to be carcinogenic, producing bladder cancer in rats. Most people also mistakenly think that these calorie-free substances will help them achieve their weight-loss goals, yet no studies demonstrate that artificial sweeteners make any difference at all in weight management. Next time you're in the mood for something sweet, enjoy apples, cherries, or grapes. Once you retool your palate, these good-for-you treats will taste as good as candy!

Drink Your Celery!

High blood pressure, the plague of the modern age, is the root cause of stroke, heart disease, and kidney failure. An old Chinese remedy for this ailment is to drink celery juice, which you can create in a blender or a juicer. One to two large glasses daily can help prevent high blood pressure or restore it to normal in those already affected. In addition, celery seed is renowned for preventing gout and other types of arthritic conditions. Studies show that this stalk contains more than a dozen anti-inflammatory agents, including one called apigenin, a cox2-inhibiting compound similar to some anti-inflammatory drugs— but in a natural form, without side effects. So do as the Chinese have been doing for centuries: eat (and drink) your celery for long life.

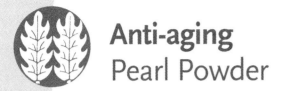

Anti-aging
Pearl Powder

The medicinal use of crushed and powdered natural pearl goes back 2,000 years in Chinese medicine. Prized by Chinese royalty for its purported anti-aging properties, pearl powder is traditionally used in herbal remedies and in ointments and massaged into the skin to prevent premature skin aging, clear surface inflammation and acne, improve vision, and calm the mind and spirit. Rich in minerals that benefit the skin, natural pearl has much more to offer than its beauty as an adornment.

Prunes'
Other Benefit

It may be a surprise to you that the prunes your grand-
mother eats on a daily basis to ease elimination are
rated by the USDA as having the highest oxygen radical
absorbence capacity (ORAC) score on the scale. The
ORAC scale was developed to assess the antioxidant
content of food: the higher the score, the better the
food's ability to neutralize cell-damaging free radicals
that lead to cancer. Raisins, blueberries, and blackberries
also score high on the ORAC scale. So incorporate
prunes into your daily diet to reap the benefits of their
cancer-preventing properties—and thank your grand-
mother for her example.

Chicory for
a Strong Heart

Chicory is a vegetable eaten in China and parts of Europe. In the United States the root is more commonly roasted and brewed as a coffee substitute. Chicory contains a compound called inulin that has been found to be useful in preventing and treating congestive heart failure. One study of its regulatory effect on the heart showed that chicory can slow a rapid heartbeat, the same function performed by the drug digitalis. It also helps lower cholesterol and slow the progression of hardening of the arteries, according to other research. So in addition to eating a low-fat, high-fiber diet and leading an active lifestyle, drink chicory tea to keep your heart pumping strong.

Asparagus Spears: Natural Weapons Against Aging

Tasty asparagus packs a punch when it comes to anti-aging functions. It is rich in potassium and vitamin A as well as folate, an important protection against cancer. Studies have also shown that asparagus is an effective preventive as well as treatment for urinary tract infections and kidney stones. Asparagus is very high in glutathione, an amino acid compound with potent antioxidant properties that is known as a cancer fighter and aging deterrent. Chinese asparagus root, a close cousin to the asparagus found on Western dinner tables, has been used to promote longevity for over two thousand years.

Hunza Fountain
of Youth Revealed.

The lifestyle of the famously long-lived Hunza discovered in the Himalaya mountains confirmed much common wisdom: they were active farmers, enjoyed an unpolluted environment, ate a largely vegetarian diet, and lived harmonious lives, seeking neither luxury nor excitement and valuing community and family. Less well known to the public is the role of one of their staple foods, apricots. Research shows that apricots possess the highest levels and widest variety of carotenoids of any food. Carotenoids are antioxidants that help prevent heart disease, reduce "bad cholesterol" levels, and protect against cancer.

Apricot kernels, according to Chinese medicine, tone the respiratory system, cure coughs and asthma, and contain high levels of essential fatty acids. One caution about apricot kernel: the tip holds a concentration of the chemical laetrile, which can cause upset to the system. To reap their benefits safely, remove the tips of the seeds before eating and limit your intake to five a day.

The Rule of 5:
Aging with Flying Colors

For thousands of years Chinese medicine has observed that there are five elemental energies in our universe as well as within our bodies (see Who You Are). These energies are represented by wood, fire, earth, metal, and water. Each of these symbols also corresponds to a color. Wood corresponds to green, fire to red, earth to yellow and orange, metal to white, and water to black, blue, and purple. According to the *Yellow Emperor's Classic of Medicine*, health and longevity depend on a balance of all five elemental energies. It recommends a diet that includes the five elemental energies every day. For each category of food you must eat all the corresponding colors. So, for example, your daily vegetables should include something green, something red, and so on. Your daily fruit, nut, bean, and grain intake should each contain all five colors as well.

Rule of 5:
The Vegetable Rainbow

To achieve a balance of the five elemental energies (see page 75), try to eat vegetables representing all of them, every day. For green (wood), your choices range from asparagus to the dark leafy greens such as spinach, broccoli, and kale. For red (fire), eat hot red peppers, red bell peppers, or beets. Vegetables in the yellow/orange group (earth) include pumpkins, squash, and yams. White vegetables (metal) could be cauliflower, jícama, or daikon radish. On the dark end of the spectrum (water), enjoy eggplant, seaweed, or black mushrooms.

Rule of 5:
Fruit and Nuts

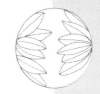

Your dietary color spectrum should also include the full variety of fruits and nuts. For green opt for lime or melon among the fruits, pumpkin seeds or pistachios in the nuts-and-seeds category. Red fruit choices might be apples, tomatoes, or cherries; for a red nut, eat pecans. In the yellow/orange group, eat papaya, mangoes, or oranges for your fruit, almonds and cashews for nuts. White fruit includes pears and bananas; white nuts are pine nuts and macadamias. Lastly, eat blueberries, blackberries, raisins, and figs for your dark-colored fruit, and chestnuts, walnuts, and black sesame for the seed group.

Rule of 5:
Beans and Grains

The rule of five also applies to beans and grains in the elemental colors. Eat from each bean group and each grain group daily. Green: lentils and mung beans; rye as your grain. Red: adzuki beans, red lentils, and red beans; buckwheat and amaranth as grains. Yellow/orange: chickpeas (garbanzo beans) and butter beans; corn and millet. White: soy beans and white beans; rice and barley. Dark: black beans and navy beans; quinoa, black wild rice. Follow the Yellow Emperor's advice in every category and you'll be consuming close to 600 carotenoids, powerful antioxidants that mop up free radicals to prevent cancer and help you see, smell, and hear better.

CHAPTER 2: How You Heal:
Herbs, Remedies, and Elixirs

In my studies of long-lived individuals and cultures around the world, the Chinese centenarians had a unique edge because they incorporated a variety of tonic herbs into their diet. These herbal practices were handed down from the Yellow Emperor through the Chinese Taoists, the earliest anti-aging scientists in the world. They served not only to maintain health and vigor but to combat disease.

The healing properties of plants are well established in the West now, after centuries of being relegated to the domain of old wives' tales. The botanical origins of many common pharmaceuticals, however, tend to be little known: How many of us are aware, for example, that the active ingredient in aspirin was discovered in white willow bark, which had been used traditionally for pain relief long before its use in chemical form? Or that the modern anticoagulant coumadin, used to prevent blood clots, originally came from turmeric?

This chapter offers tips on staying fit and fighting illness by natural means, with everything from dietary supplements that remove carcinogens from your body to tonic herbal elixirs with energizing properties. These are nature's gifts: use them wisely to live long.

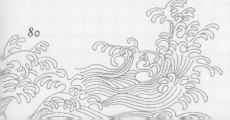

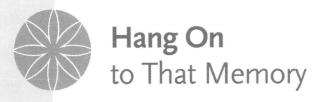

Hang On
to That Memory

Phosphatidylserine (PS) is a well-documented nutrient
used in Europe to reverse age-related dementia and
memory loss. PS is a compound made naturally by the
body, and studies have shown that it lowers one's stress
response. Apparently PS boosts various neurotransmitters
in the brain that activate reasoning, concentration, and
memory. That means PS increases one's ability to with-
stand the harmful effects of stress on one's body.

Unstress
Your Heart

In Europe, Japan, and Israel, coenzyme Q-10 is a popular supplementary treatment for various heart conditions. The compound is a powerful antioxidant that occurs naturally in all the cells of the body and helps the heart function more efficiently during times of stress. Due to its importance in cellular energy production, it is an essential nutrient for degenerative conditions, fatigue, and muscle weakness. Co-Q10 has also been found to prevent premature aging of the skin.

The Yellow Cure
for Sluggish Blood

Did you know that the anticoagulant medication coumadin
was originally extracted from turmeric? This yellow-colored
spice, perhaps best recognized for the taste it adds to
curry blends, has been used in Asia for its medicinal properties for many centuries. Turmeric is traditionally used as
a blood activator, a pain reliever for joints, and a liver and
gall bladder cleanser. Studies show its benefits for prevention of blood clots, reducing inflammation, increasing bile
secretion, lowering cholesterol, and possibly preventing
certain cancers. If you are taking coumadin, also called
warfarin, you should avoid turmeric so levels in your
bloodstream will not get too high. But for the rest, keep
the flow going by using turmeric in food or taking it as
a supplement.

Speed Up
Fat Metabolism

An amino acid manufactured in your liver, L-carnitine helps facilitate fat metabolism, increases energy production in muscle cells, promotes fat loss, and increases circulation in the brain. The substance also helps reduce triglycerides and increase good cholesterol, thereby protecting the heart. Because it also prevents fat oxidation in the brain, it shows some promise in preventing Alzheimer's and Parkinson's diseases. Rich sources of L-carnitine include meats, fish, poultry, wheat, avocado, milk, and fermented soybeans.

Nature's
Pollution-Fighter

The powerful antioxidant and detoxifier L-cysteine can help protect your body from the harmful effects of pollution, heavy metals, chemicals, radiation, alcohol, and smoke. This naturally occurring amino acid may also help boost the immune system, protect against heart disease, build muscle, and decrease fat buildup. L-cysteine is also useful for combatting inflammation and promoting healthy hair and nail growth. The substance is found in eggs, fish, almonds, sesame seeds, soy, pumpkin seeds, peanuts, legumes, avocados, bananas, whole grains, and brewer's yeast.

Blood Sugar
Balancing Act

Chromium performs a variety of important functions to keep us healthy: it helps to stabilize blood sugar levels, metabolize amino acids and fats, and lower bad cholesterol while increasing the good. These properties make it useful in controlling diabetes and hypoglycemia and preventing cardiovascular disease. Chromium, however, is a difficult mineral to absorb, as most of it is eliminated through the bowels and kidneys. As you get older, your body stores less and less of the mineral, which may be why age is a risk factor for diabetes, the third leading cause of death in the United States. Foods rich in chromium include brewer's yeast, broccoli, beets, legumes, mushrooms, nuts, whole wheat, black pepper, blackstrap molasses, meat, and cheese. Since you only need trace amounts of chromium, a dietary supplement of 100 to 200 micrograms daily will do the job.

Versatile ALA
Combats Alzheimer's

Alpha-lipoic acid (ALA) plays the key role of converting our food into cellular energy. ALA is a very special compound because, unlike other antioxidants, which only work in either water or fatty environments, this one functions in both. When the body uses up vitamins C and E during times of stress, ALA converts the by-products into new antioxidant compounds, thus "recycling" the vitamins. Alpha-lipoic acid prevents the type of nerve damage seen in diabetes and aging-related ailments such as Parkinson's and Alzheimer's diseases; it also helps ward off cancer, cardiovascular disease, cataracts, and diabetes.

The Mother of All
Hormones: DHEA

DHEA (dehydroepiandrosterone) is the most abundant steroid in the human body. Because it can generate so many hormones in response to our bodies' needs, it is often considered the mother of all hormones. And like a good mother, DHEA protects and supports us in numerous ways. It is a potent immunity booster, yet also helps to control autoimmune disorders, in which the immune system mistakenly attacks the body's own tissue. It has also been shown to possess powerful anticancer properties and to prevent DNA damage such as UV effects on the skin. The steroid helps protect against arteriosclerosis, lowers blood pressure, reduces inflammation in the brain, prevents fat accumulation, and improves heart function. Maintaining a sufficient level of DHEA can slow much aging-related degeneration, but because it is a hormonal precursor, anyone suffering from hormone imbalance should consult a doctor before taking it in supplement form. Better yet, eat lots of sweet potatoes and yams for their rich, plant-source DHEA, and your body will be able to sort out its needs.

DNA
in a Pill

The wear and tear of aging depletes your storehouse of
nucleic acids, which are the building blocks of DNA and
RNA in every cell of your body. Replenishing your stock of
these nutrients may slow down the aging process. Animal
studies and limited clinical observations with humans
have shown promise for increased life span and other
quality-of-health measurements such as increased energy,
healthier skin, and reduction in age spots. You can now
take nucleic acids in supplement form or simply load up
on nucleic acid—rich foods such as sardines, mushrooms,
asparagus, wheat germ, salmon, and spinach.

Anti-Aging Herb with a 5,000-Year Track Record

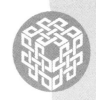

Panax ginseng is perhaps the world's best-known herb. Popularly employed to increase energy and stamina, it has been used medically in Asia for more than 5,000 years. In China, ginseng is more valuable than gold due to its seemingly miraculous properties of restoring health. The name *panax* is related to the word *panacea*, which means "cure-all." Scientists in the West have confirmed ginseng's efficacy in various traditional uses. Commonly considered an "adaptogen," ginseng enhances body functions and the immune system to help people adapt to the negative effects of physical and environmental stress. Ginseng helps improve coordination and reaction time as well as increase endurance and decrease fatigue. It boosts energy gently, rather than stimulating the central nervous system, as coffee does. There is also strong evidence that ginseng can help the body fight off infection, protect liver and heart health, normalize cholesterol and blood sugar levels, regulate the function of hormones, and improve memory and cognitive functions. People taking ginseng often report overall improvement in well-being. Thanks to widespread cultivation and abundant supply, this truly remarkable anti-aging herb is available to and affordable for people all over the world.

Think Best
with Low Stress

A prized berry that has been used for thousands of years to rejuvenate and revitalize the senses, schisandra contains several vitamins and flavonoids that possess antioxidant and immune-boosting properties. It is considered an energy tonic that enhances both physical endurance and mental concentration and at the same time soothes the nerves, taking the edge off anxiety. As a beauty treatment, schisandra is said to promote radiant skin tone. It has been used as an adjunct support for immune function in patients undergoing chemotherapy and helps to protect the liver and kidneys. Grown in Asia, schisandra is available as a supplement from health food stores.

Natural Boost
for Growth Hormone

Lycium berry, also known as wolfberry, is a delicious fruit native to Asia that has long been known for its tonic effects, especially on vision and the brain. Lycium berry contains polysaccharides, which stimulate the immune system and signal the pituitary to secrete human growth hormone. A good source of vitamins B and C, zinc, calcium, germanium, selenium, phosphorus, and other trace minerals, lycium also has the highest concentration of carotenoids, especially beta-carotene, of any plant in the world and is thus a powerful antioxidant. The berry is traditionally used together with other Chinese tonic herbs to increase sexual potency and fertility. A wonderful feature of lycium is that it is safe to use, with no known side effects. The health-giving berries also taste good—use them instead of raisins in cereals and trail mix.

Mobilize Your Body to Fight Off Flu

Astragalus has been used in Asia for more than 2,000 years to strengthen vitality and prevent illness, especially colds and flu. It has been found to stimulate the body's own production of interferon, a powerful immune protein that increases your ability to fight infectious disease. Astragalus restores healthy immune function despite physical, chemical, or radiation damage. Cancer patients taking astragalus during chemotherapy and radiation treatments tend to have far fewer side effects and recover at a faster rate. The herb is also beneficial for the skin and speeds the healing of wounds and infections on the body's surface. Of side interest, it can also increase sperm production and motility, helpful in treating male infertility. This wonderful addition to your natural anti-aging medicine cabinet increases the longevity of human cells and has no known toxicity.

Hail to the Queen Bee!

In Asian cultures, royal jelly is regarded as a longevity tonic that enhances energy, virility, and immunity. Rich in vitamins and collagen, royal jelly is used to feed queen bees. When given the same diet as the worker bees, a queen bee lives the same life span, seven to eight weeks. In nature, however, the queen bee is fed exclusively on royal jelly—and lives for five to seven years! Royal jelly also fights tumors, especially the sarcoma type. An anti-bacterial protein in the substance, dubbed *royalisin*, is effective against certain bacteria, including streptococcus and staphylococcus. Royal jelly is available in supplement form from herb shops and health food stores.

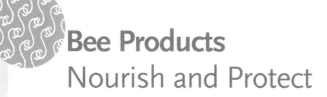

Bee Products
Nourish and Protect

Two bee products that may surprise you with their benefits are bee pollen and propolis. Bee pollen contains a rich supply of vitamins, minerals, enzymes, and amino acids. It protects the liver from toxins, benefits men with enlarged prostates, and boosts energy and vitality.

The bees use propolis, consisting mainly of tree resins, to seal cracks in hives and act as a protective layer against invading microbes and other organisms. It is rich in flavonoids with both antioxidant and anti-inflammatory properties. Propolis also contains terpenoids that possess antibacterial, antiviral, antifungal, and antiprotozoan agents. Like some prescription antibiotics, it prevents bacterial cell division and breaks down the invading organism's cell walls and cytoplasm. The substance is available in capsules or in propolis-enriched honey. To nourish and protect, what works for bees works for humans, too!

Chinese Athletes'
Secret Energizer

Cordyceps has received quite a bit of attention since the news broke that record-breaking Chinese Olympic runners use it to vastly increase their performance. The mushroom's energizing properties have been prized in the East for thousands of years, but it was in relatively short supply until modern advances in growing techniques made it more widely available to consumers. The same vitality-enhancing properties that aid athletes to achieve feats of strength and endurance can help you live longer: cordyceps helps increase cellular energy metabolism, boosts adrenal functions to adapt to stress, modulates immune function, increases capillary circulation, and improves oxygen utilization.

Brain-Shaped Herb
Keeps You Smart

The leaf of the ginkgo tree is shaped like the human brain, and some say this is why, in Asia, it has always been reputed to benefit mental processes. Ginkgo, one of the most studied plants, has been confirmed to boost circulation to the brain and other organs, improving memory and cognitive functions. In addition, ginkgo has been widely used as a longevity tonic in Asia and Europe. The leaf, in teas and herbal extracts, is the best-known and most commonly available form, but ginkgo nut, used in the culinary traditions of China and Japan, also has therapeutic properties and is said to strengthen lung function.

Hawthorn for
a Brawny Heart

Widely used since the seventeenth century by European herbalists, hawthorn was traditionally considered a digestive aid for heavy meats and rich foods as well as a potent activator of the circulatory system. Recent European studies of this bioflavonoid-rich plant have confirmed its cardiovascular benefits, including lowering blood pressure during exertion, strengthening the heart muscle, and improving blood flow to the heart and throughout the body. Additionally, hawthorn has been found to lower cholesterol and balance blood sugar. As a beverage or a supplement, hawthorn is indispensable in your arsenal against aging.

Botanical
Detoxifiers

To give our cells the best chance of functioning smoothly to keep us young, we need to remove toxins that accumulate in the body. Nature has given us plants that possess potent cleansing properties. Some work by helping the liver detoxify; others cause toxins to be excreted from the bowels and urinary tract. A traditional formula for internal cleansing consists of chrysanthemum flower, mint, cassia seed, and dandelion to help cleanse the liver and clear the head; hawthorn berry to clear the arteries of fats and cholesterol; and cocklebur fruit, which opens the sinuses and expels mucus. To keep toxins and pollutants from building up to dangerous levels in your body, make it a regular practice to consume cleansing herbs and to fast for brief periods.

Native American
Power Herb

The herb known by the Latin name ligusticum has many varieties around the world: Native Americans call it osha; the Chinese species is named chuan xiong. It has long been a key herb in the longevity tradition of China, prized for its powers to boost the immune system, activate blood circulation, and relieve pain. Studies confirm ligusticum's efficacy in preventing stroke and restoring blood flow to the brain and heart, and the herb has been found to inhibit tumor growth in animals. Used along with other immune-support herbs during chemotherapy or to treat anemia, ligusticum is often taken in a supplement blend for synergistic effects.

Natural Vitamins,
Not Petrochemical Pills

Many health seekers take vitamins and minerals by the handful every day in the belief that they are effective health aids. Often, because of the dietary supplements' low bioavailability—the absorption factor—what people consume is excreted from the bladder and bowels without being metabolized. Many vitamins are synthetic, made from petrochemicals that have very little biological activity. The supplements with the highest bioavailability use extracts from organic, whole foods. The best way to take vitamins and minerals is in the form of powdered or liquid concentrates or oils made from bee pollen, barley, wheat grass, kelp, spirulina, chlorophyll, brewer's yeast, bonemeal, wheat germ, flax, and fish oils. Of course, by eating a nutritious and varied diet rich in whole foods, you will absorb these nutrients the way nature intended.

Fenugreek
Foments Vitality

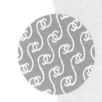

Long known as a vitality enhancer in Chinese medicine, fenugreek is traditionally used to boost low energy, promote recovery from serious illness, and improve poor sexual function. Recent studies have found fenugreek to be helpful in reducing harmful LDL cholesterol and taming blood sugar in diabetics. Its beneficial effects may be due to its content of phytosterols—plant hormones that mimic body hormones essential for health maintenance. Fenugreek can be found in health food stores or herb shops.

Saw Palmetto
for a Healthier Prostate

Declining hormone levels in aging men can lead to
swollen prostate and waning libido. Chronic prostate
problems can cause constricted, frequent urinary flow
and may result in prostate cancer, the second most common type of cancer in men. Saw palmetto is an herb that
has been traditionally used for easing prostate concerns.
Studies have shown that it balances testosterone levels,
reduces inflammation, and provides an abundance of
essential fatty acids. It can also be helpful for menopausal
women when hormonal changes result in increased body
hair. Saw palmetto is widely available in health food stores.

Secrets of
Chinese Women

Throughout China and Asia, angelica root, or dong quai, has been maintaining women's health for thousands of years. It is traditionally used to regulate menstrual periods, enhance fertility, build blood, strengthen bones, and maintain healthy hair, skin, and nails. It also relieves hot flashes and other symptoms related to menopausal changes. But studies have shown that in addition to reducing these discomforts, dong quai increases immune function and reduces levels of damaging free radicals in the bloodstream. Could this be why so many Chinese women live to an advanced age?

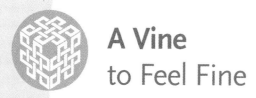

A Vine
to Feel Fine

Gynostemma is a vine that grows wild in the southwestern regions of China and has been used traditionally as a heart tonic and energy booster. Studies have shown that it may help to lower cholesterol, blood pressure, and heart rate. Gynostemma is also rich in antioxidants, containing more than eighty saponins that help prevent cancer and increase immune functions. It is available as a tea or in supplement form.

A Whale of a Bargain
for Protein

Do you ever wonder how whales grow to their huge size
from eating only single-cell organisms called plankton,
the tiny plants and animals floating in the ocean? The type
of plankton suitable for human consumption consists of
microalgae with names like chlorella and spirulina, which
are by far the highest source of protein of any food in
nature. One teaspoon of microalgae contains as much
protein as one ounce of beef. The chlorophyll in microalgae also cleanses and detoxifies the body.

Soldiers' Miracle Herb
to Heal Wounds

With aging, it is more important than ever to avoid loss of blood of any kind, from accidental wounds, surgery, or conditions of internal bleeding. This puts stress on the system to replace the blood and, in the last case, to move the excess fluid at the hemorrhage site—not to mention inducing temporary anemia, which can affect many parts of the body. The active ingredient in Chinese medicine's most celebrated remedies, yunnan bai yao, is tian qi or pseudoginseng, which was carried by soldiers on the battlefield to be used in case of bullet wounds. Although it is used topically in powdered form, it is also effective taken internally as a tincture or in capsules.

Ancient Formula
Strengthens Your Essence

According to Chinese longevity philosophy, *jing*, or
essence, is the basic substance of life. Innate essence
is inherited from parentage and can be refined through
practices such as tai chi, qigong, and meditation, while
a second kind of jing, acquired during your life, can be
replenished through diet, nutrition, and longevity herbs.
A formula for enduring youth passed down in our family
medical tradition contains such essence-building herbs
as Chinese wild yam, ligustri fruit, schisandra berry,
sesame seed, eucommia bark, *ho shou wu* (*fo ti*) root,
and cistanches root. Studies of all these plants confirm
their positive effects on the hormonal, immune, and
metabolic systems.

May the Life Force
Be with You

Qi, or life force, determines your energy level and optimum function. Thinking, working, and playing all require and consume qi from your body. Traditional Chinese culture understands the need for energy replenishment. Plants and herbs such as lotus seed, china root, longan fruit, pearl barley, ginseng, and fox nut have long been successfully used to strengthen digestion and boost qi.

Nutrition
for the Spirit

Shen, or spirit, is the consciousness that animates your
being. Your life would be meaningless and unfulfilling
without spirit, even though your physical body could
survive for years until death. Therefore your spirit needs
nurturing, just as your body does, through self-love, discipline, and spirit-nourishing herbs. For example, bamboo
shaving is traditionally used to strengthen objectivity and
dispel undue worry. Lily bulb restores joy and eases sadness. Dragon bone maintains stability and lessens anger
and depression. Chinese senega root promotes clarity and
calms excessive excitement and anxiety. Rehmannia root
strengthens will and dispels fear. All are available in
Chinese herb shops and your local acupuncturist's office.

Spring Back
After Surgery

If you should have to undergo major surgery, you can greatly improve your chances for a swift recovery and many more years of life. Here's how: Go to your acupuncturist for a weekly "tune-up," starting four weeks before surgery, to ready your body for rapid healing. Stop taking ginkgo and vitamin E three weeks before the operation, and do not resume until 10 days afterward. These substances have an anticoagulant effect and can slow your body's repair of the incision. Just before you enter the operating room, place five grains of homeopathic arnica under your tongue. (If you are receiving general anesthetic you will be told not to eat or drink, but these tiny, dissolving granules do not violate that prohibition.) As soon as you awaken, take five more. Arnica helps the body recover from the trauma of being opened with a scalpel.

"Bone Up"
After a Stroke

There is no reason why stroke victims cannot fully recover and live long lives—assuming they know how to take the best care possible. An often unrecognized side effect of a stroke is lowered bone density, especially on the side that was more affected by the stroke. A study of post-stroke patients showed decreased levels of vitamin D_3 and an increased risk of hip fractures. The group given D_3 showed significantly improved bone mineral density over the untreated group and had fewer fractures. To avoid a broken hip—recovering from which is another arduous task that can debilitate your body's healing mechanisms— take vitamin D_3 supplements if you suffer a stroke.

Velvet
Regeneration

Chinese medicine always looks to nature for a model of desired health effects. Eastern practitioners long ago took note of the fact that stags lose their antlers every year and then quickly regenerate them. They soon recognized that velvet deer antler (VDA, meaning antlers in the growth stage, before they calcify into horn) was a potent rejuvenator and growth tonic. Its traditional uses are to treat age-related impotence, lower back pain, and fatigue. Western studies confirm that VDA stimulates the body's production of IGF-1, which is the substance that cells make from human growth hormone. VDA's regenerative characteristics have been put to work to increase mental powers, stimulate blood circulation to the brain, improve eyesight, and aid in arthritis relief. It can be found in supplement form at health food stores and Chinese pharmacies.

Primo Amino
for Mood

No one can live long without the will to go on, and mood swings can sometimes make us feel that life is too much for us. These episodes are often due to inner imbalances or deficiencies. The Europeans use supplements of a natural compound found in human cells to regulate mood and restore a healthy outlook. SAMe (S-adenosyl-L-methionine) is produced from methionine, an amino acid that plays a role in the production of "upside" neurotransmitters such as dopamine and serotonin. One study showed that SAMe worked on patients who had had no success with conventional antidepressants. Other clinical tests indicate the substance can also alleviate osteoarthritis and help repair the liver. To get a boost from SAMe, take a supplement combining it with vitamins B_6 and B_{12}. It will remind you of what you already know: life is worth it!

Fight Fatal Disorders
with Folic Acid

It's impossible to predict who will contract a fatal age-related disorder such as Parkinson's or Alzheimer's disease, but we can lower our odds by keeping an eye on the current data. Scientists have observed that older people tend to be deficient in folate, which enables vitamins B_6 and B_{12} to aid in hormone secretion, synthesize DNA, and manufacture the protective coating around nerves. All three tasks are thought to be major elements in our bodies' defenses against these diseases. Folate is found in numerous foods, including spinach, kale, beet greens, chard, Brussels sprouts, asparagus, and broccoli—but it is destroyed by heat, so they must be eaten raw. This is one case in which the synthetic form, folic acid, is more easily absorbed by the body than the natural one. A dose of 800 micrograms per day is recommended for people over 50.

Be Proactive
with Probiotics

Most people in the United States have occasionally
had recourse to antibiotics, a key player in the Western
model of fighting disease. Let's think about the word:
anti means "against"; *bios* means "life." An antibiotic
destroys small organisms within our bodies, without
distinguishing between the beneficial ones, such as
intestinal bacteria, and the damaging invaders. This is
one reason that diarrhea is a frequent side effect of
antibiotics. Taking a supplement of lactobacillus—a
probiotic, or promoter of "good" bacteria—will restore
the healthy organisms needed to digest our food. That's
not all: lactobacillus inhibits the growth of H. Pylori, the
microbe responsible for up to 90 percent of stomach
ulcers. And ulcers never helped anyone live to a ripe
old age!

Sage Advice
on Angina

If you experience pain and constriction in the chest and neck, especially on the left side, see a doctor at once: these are symptoms of angina, a serious heart condition. Chinese medicine looks at angina as a stagnation of energy in the heart. You'll want to take strong measures right away, especially stopping smoking and eliminating animal fats from your diet. It's time to set a long-range plan for heart health. From now on your lifestyle should include regular exercise, plenty of fiber in your diet, eating oily fish, and lessening stress however you can.

To treat angina, the traditional Chinese prescription is to chop one red sage root into chunks and boil briefly, no longer than eight minutes. (Be sure to use the kind of sage that has red leaves; green-leaf sage will not have the same effect.) Drink the liquid as tea sweetened with honey. Cinnamon twigs, safflower, and red peony, found in Chinese herb shops and some health food stores, are also of help.

Herbal Help
for Hepatitis

Long-lifers need good livers—that goes without saying. The liver plays the crucial role of filtering toxins in the body, but when you're hit with viral hepatitis it falls down on the job. Symptoms may include severe fatigue, nausea, aching muscles, and jaundice, and it can take months to recover. Milk thistle seeds help damaged liver cells to rebuild. Crush one teaspoonful of seeds, cover with one cup of water, and let stand for 10 minutes before drinking. Repeat three times a day. Dandelion eaten raw is another potent member of the rescue team; ginseng and licorice can help restore failing energy.

The big gun is oriental wormwood, which can be taken fresh or in capsule form. Before taking this potent herb, consult a doctor of Chinese medicine, who will determine the right dose for you.

Let Nature Help You
Stop Smoking

When you embark on your longevity program, you may find it best to start by implementing the easier changes in diet, lifestyle, and surroundings. As you become more serious about your goal, you'll want to stop smoking tobacco. Your first step should be to examine each impulse to reach for a cigarette: Is it habit? Stress? A physical craving? Use meditation and the other anti-stress tips in this book to start addressing the origins of this urge. When you feel your resolve is strong, you can cleanse your body of nicotine using a combination of herbal aids that help to rebalance your body chemistry. Gardenia, gotu kola, sarsaparilla, gentian, and licorice root are a few of nature's botanical supports for your efforts. Such formulas are available in health food stores.

Make the Thyroid
Fly Right

The thyroid is the pacemaker for the metabolism. The little gland in the neck uses iodine, which controls the rate of activity in the body's cells. An overactive thyroid (hyperthyroidism) can cause palpitations, sweating, weight loss, and bulging eyes; an underactive one (hypothyroidism) may result in weight gain, lethargy, hair loss, and excessive sleeping. If yours gets hyper, drink an infusion of bugleweed to lessen palpitations, and consume fritillary bulb in liquid concentrate or tablets. Acupuncture may also help lessen overproduction of thyroid hormones. If it's hypo, on the other hand, consume seaweed, as food or supplements to restore balance, and engage in aerobic exercise to stimulate the gland's hormone production.

"Fat Vitamins"
Ward Off Breast Cancer

Essential fatty acids are like fat vitamins, if you will, that are used in making cell membranes. They are also important in the body's ability to reduce inflammation and prevent the many degenerative diseases associated with it. Studies show that women with a high intake of essential fatty acids (EFAs) are at much lower risk of developing breast cancer. Dietary sources of EFAs are flaxseed, borage, walnut, and hemp seed oils. You can consume these oils on salads and in smoothies, or simply take a tablespoon daily as a supplement. Of course, make sure you're getting your EFAs from cold-pressed, organic oil.

Control Yeast to Maintain
Good Body Ecology

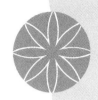

Yeast infections are a pain, as most women can attest, but the yeast organism can be more insidious than in this easily treatable vaginal ailment. It often reproduces unnoticed inside your body until its population is out of control. Eating a diet overloaded with sugar, white flour, and fermented foods encourages chronic overproliferation of yeast. This contributes to malabsorption of food and eventually malnutrition if the body ecology is not restored to normal.

To combat internal yeast, eliminate white flour, sugar, fats, and processed foods from your diet. Eat only whole grains and vegetables, adding natural antifungal substances such as citrus seed extract, caprylic acid, and garlic supplements, all available in health food stores. Additionally, repopulating your intestinal environment with acidophilus supplements or plain goat's yogurt over a course of three to four months will gradually readjust the balance of organisms within your body.

Hope for
Ex-alcoholics

Don't feel you have no prospects for longevity if your body has been ravaged by alcoholism in the past. Chinese traditional medicine uses natural substances to treat cirrhosis of the liver with great success. Three herbs are especially effective in helping to regenerate this vital organ: Eclipta (*han lian cao*) is a liver tonic, antifungal, and anti-inflammatory herb. Bupleurum root (*chai hu*), used as a treatment for an enlarged or chemically damaged liver as well as for hepatitis, may be taken in capsule or tincture form. Milk thistle (Sylibum marianum) improves liver function in patients with cirrhosis. All these herbs can be taken as a tincture or tea by itself, or as part of a personalized formula. Always consult a trained herbalist for dosage of these powerful herbs.

Call Nature's "Fire" Fighters

Inflammation in the body resembles fire in its destructive power. Recent research strongly indicates that inflammation is the root of all degenerative diseases like heart disease, arthritis, Alzheimer's, Parkinson's, and senility. The most severe of these conditions are incurable and fatal. But nature's inflammation fighter comes to the rescue. Fruits such as papaya, pineapple, and kiwi contain an anti-inflammatory enzyme called bromelain that can reduce the inflammatory process, modulate overactive immune responses that cause it, and relieve allergies. So before you resort to an anti-inflammatory drug, try eating copious amounts of papaya, pineapple, and kiwi. Add cherries and grapes, which are rich in phytochemicals that also fight inflammation.

Western Meds
Can Leave You Dead

It's no wonder that more and more people are turning to alternative practices such as acupuncture. One study shows that the side effects of pharmaceutical drugs kill some 140,000 people in the United States each year and cost the country over $136 billion annually. These numbers don't count addictions and suicides—the side effects alone of prescribed drugs are the nation's fifth leading cause of death. Herb-related deaths amount to fewer than 50 a year, according to 10 years of statistics and research. The majority of herbs on the marketplace are safe, effective substitutes for drug medications. For example, saw palmetto capsules can replace Proscar, a drug used to reduce the symptoms of an enlarged prostate in men. Valerian tea is an herbal substitute for sleeping pills, which are often addictive. Frankincense in tincture or tablet form serves as an effective natural anti-inflammatory to replace nonsteroid anti-inflammatory agents, which cause gastric distress. If you are concerned about your long-term quality of health and length of life, seek out a doctor who is knowledgeable about alternative remedies and discuss natural, plant-based alternative remedies to your current medication.

Live Long—
Without Arthritis

More than 40 million Americans, one out of six, have
some form of arthritis—but you don't have to be one of
them. Recent studies show that osteoarthritis is not an
inevitable part of the aging process. Here's your program:
maintain ideal weight; get regular low-impact exercise; eat
a diet rich in antioxidants such as vitamins C, A, and E;
get some sun for vitamin D; eat lots of enzyme-rich foods
containing bromelain, like papaya and pineapples; take
supplements such as glucosamine and chondroitin that
support joint and cartilage health; and use the herbs ginger, turmeric, and cinnamon, all of which can help reduce
inflammation and increase circulation. Additionally, some
people may find it helpful to avoid foods from the night-
shade family, which contain a plant alkaloid called sola-
nine. These include tomatoes, potatoes, eggplants, and
bell peppers.

From the
Horse's Mouth

One of the most common circulatory problems encountered as we age is the weakening of our blood vessels, particularly veins. Varicose veins are a frequent result. As usual, nature can help: horse chestnut, a favorite weed for horses to munch on (hence its name), is a traditional remedy and preventive against varicose veins, spider veins, and broken capillaries. It strengthens the vascular system by toning up the vein walls, easing the flow of blood back to the heart. Horse chestnut prevents vein enlargement and has been found to be as effective as support stockings in reducing lower leg swelling. Horse chestnut capsules are widely available in health food stores.

Gone with the Wind

Common colds and flus can turn into serious respiratory diseases such as pneumonia, which claims many lives among the elderly. Eastern medicine sees colds and flus as "wind" disorders. A famous remedy in Chinese medicine to prevent or dispel invasive wind consists of astragalus root, siler root (*fang feng*), schisandra berries, and atractylodes (*bai zhu*). Western medicine calls them adaptogens, which increase the body's defense mechanisms and help the immune system work better in times of stress. They can be found separately in health food stores or in a formula called Jade Screen in Chinese pharmacies. In addition, wash your hands frequently with soap and water and inhale vapors from eucalyptus, oregano, and lavender teas, which are antibacterial, antiviral, and decongesting.

Natural Pain Relief
Has a Role in Longevity

Pain, especially chronic pain, is the number one reason that people refrain from exercise. Yet exercise is critical to one's longevity. Your healing plan should include treatments to resolve the underlying cause of the pain as well as an effective pain remedy. White willow bark contains salicin, a compound found in aspirin—in fact, aspirin was originally discovered in and extracted from this bark. Besides its pain-relieving property, white willow bark is an anticoagulant, which helps prevent formation of blood clots and thickening of blood that can lead to heart attacks and strokes. A major advantage of using willow bark over its pharmaceutical cousin, aspirin, is that it does not cause gastric upset and erode the stomach lining.

Women's "Second Spring"

In Chinese culture we call menopause the "second spring," because the end of a woman's childbearing years gives rise to a new phase of life empowered by her accumulated wisdom. Physically, however, debilitating symptoms can appear as estrogen production slows: hot flashes, insomnia, headaches, mood swings, dryness, diminished skin elasticity, memory loss. To facilitate the transition I recommend eating foods that are high in phytoestrogens, plant estrogens that are a weaker form of the body's hormone. Such foods include apples, brown rice, cabbage, carrots, beans and legumes, beets, citrus, cornmeal, oatmeal, potatoes, radish, fennel, and soy.

Soy is rich in genistein, which, like estrogen, protects against osteoporosis and other aging symptoms. Many other beans contain similar amounts of such substances: black-eyed peas, pinto beans, mung beans, adzuki beans, fava beans, northern beans, yellow split peas, red kidney beans, lima beans, and black turtle beans are all high in phytoestrogens. Additionally, regular weight-bearing cardiovascular exercise, as well as energy-based exercise forms like tai chi and yoga are essential for a flourishing second spring.

Live Long,
Last Long

The male version of menopause, called andropause, starts around 50 years of age when hormone levels decline, often resulting in diminished desire and ability to perform sexually. Additionally, most men at this age have developed a certain amount of plaque buildup in the circulatory system, which decreases blood flow to the penis. These two factors can produce erectile dysfunction, for many men the most disturbing aspect of aging.

Chinese medicine enjoys a long history of successfully reversing the decline in male sexual potency. An herbal remedy including deer antler velvet, ginseng root, morinda root, Chinese Senega root, and horny goat weed, among others, is used to increase circulation, activate testicular function, and stimulate the hormonal system. Studies show that horny goat weed has a moderate androgen-like effect and serves to stimulate the sensory nerves in the penile area. Ask for Dragon Male formula in health food stores.

I also recommend that patients with erectile dysfunction perform plenty of cardiovascular exercise, reduce stress, get adequate amounts of sleep, and eat a diet rich in zinc, which is found in oysters, pumpkin seeds, sunflower seeds, peanuts, Brazil nuts, cashews, beans and legumes, brown rice, and wheat germ. Instead of resorting to a drug like Viagra, why not try these natural methods for a healthier, longer-lasting effect?

Longevity for
the Female Libido

As aging sets in, women begin to experience a noticeable waning of their interest in sexual activity. Most of this phenomenon is due to a decline in the hormones estrogen and testosterone; contributing factors may include stress, poor self-image, fatigue, and an aging partner. To preserve and enhance the hormonal aspect of libido, I often recommend for my patients an herbal formula, Feminine Desire, to stimulate endocrine production as well as vitality, energy, and natural desires. It combines horny goat weed, which is effective for both male and female sexual potency, with herbs such as dong quai, wild yam, and ginseng, and spices like anise, ginger, and turmeric.

The Digestion Question:
3 Herbal Answers

Of the ten top-selling drugs in the United States, three are specifically for indigestion and heartburn. That's because we live in a culture marked by poor diet and digestion— and the poor health and short life span that go with it. You'll find many tips in this book for practices that can help, such as controlling your weight, eating smaller meals, chewing thoroughly, reducing stress, and avoiding coffee, cigarettes, alcohol, and deep-fried foods. In addition, taking certain common, easily available herbs on a regular basis can prevent or relieve digestive problems. Peppermint has many well-documented properties: it increases healthy gastric secretions, relaxes the intestines, soothes spasms, settles the stomach, and alleviates gas. Ginger, also extensively studied, has been shown to soothe the digestive lining and balance gastric juices. Chamomile is another excellent herb for settling the stomach. You can combine the three herbs, steep them as tea, and drink it at mealtimes.

See Yourself
at 100

In our increasingly aging population, millions of people suffer age-related eyes disorders such as glaucoma, cataracts, and macular degeneration that can lead to blindness. Nature's remedies can help you prevent vision loss. Bilberry, a cousin of blueberry, promotes blood flow to eye nerves and has been found to be a rich source of antioxidants. Other herbal agents include wolfberry, a Chinese herb traditionally used to strengthen eyesight; chrysanthemum flower, which reduces pressure buildup in the eye; and peppermint, rich in antioxidants and a traditional treatment to clear the vision. All of these may be used in supplement form if they are otherwise unavailable. Lutein, a substance found in dark green leafy vegetables, helps prevent cataracts, and a daily dose of vitamin E can cut the risk of cataract by half. Eat your carrots, of course—they're full of vitamin A—and care for your eyes by avoiding irritants, eye fatigue, and strong sunlight (or use UV-protective sunglasses).

Nature's Energizers
for Alertness

Low energy and vitality is probably the most common complaint of aging. But instead of reaching for harsh stimulants like coffee, for which you pay a price, try the potent yet gentle energizers in your spice rack. Studies have found that compounds in everyday herbs and spices can increase mental function and physical vitality. One compound in particular, cineole, has been found to enhance the ability of rats to navigate mazes. Of the herbs rich in cineole, cardamom tops the list, followed by eucalyptus, spearmint, rosemary, and ginger. So instead of that cup of java, make yourself a tea from any of these herbs to spice up your energy.

Longevity Loud
and Clear

Why does hearing wane as we age? Blood supply to the
auditory nerve diminishes, and neural conductivity to the
brain declines. Eastern medicine has long used acupuncture to increase blood flow to the auditory region and
normalize conduction, which can alleviate tinnitus (ring-
ing in the ears) as well as hearing loss. Can't find an
acupuncturist? You can take steps to improve your hearing on your own. Daily cardiovascular exercise will boost
hearing function by increasing circulation overall. The
supplement niacin, or vitamin B_3, helps dilate capillaries,
promoting blood flow to the tiny blood vessels in the
inner ear that feed the nerve. Another B vitamin, choline,
is essential for the body to produce a key neurotransmit-
ter, acetylcholine. Good sources of niacin and choline
include legumes and beans, especially soy beans, wheat
germ, whole grains, avocado, brewer's yeast, peanuts,
leafy greens, and fish.

Chapter 3: Where You Are:
Environment, Ecology, and Community

From the rugged mountains of Armenia to the verdant valleys of Ecuador, the pristine foothills of the Himalayas to the tranquil island of Okinawa, it is no accident that centenarians live in clusters around the world. These Shangri-las all share common characteristics—clean air, good water, low stress, tight communities, and unspoiled nature. When it comes to longevity, environment is half of the equation.

Most people of the world must contend with the side effects of modern progress: the assaults of pollution and toxins. Science and technological progress have improved conveniences, hygiene, and medical care, contributing to increases in overall life expectancy around the world. But the gains in quality and length of life are being derailed by the toxic by-products of our very own industrial prowess.

Fundamental to achieving exceptional health is harmony with your environment. Not only have we made our environment cancerous for ourselves, but we have also made it harder for other organisms in nature to thrive. Since the beginning of the Industrial Revolution, hundreds of thousands of species have vanished from our planet due to human activities. But if we don't heed the warning signs, we may eventually extinguish ourselves. That wouldn't do much for your longevity goals.

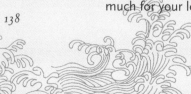

Harmonizing with our environment also applies to the subtle spheres. The energies that crisscross the surface of our planet have long been recognized by the Chinese sages. This interplay—invisible but with a powerful influence on our health, well-being, and success in life—is called feng shui, literally meaning "wind and water." Similar to the practice of restoring flow to the body's energy meridians in acupuncture, alignment of your living and working environment with earth's meridians will bring a positive energy flow into your life.

Your environment includes your community. The human milieu in which you work and live plays a role in the success of your life-extension plan. Your community can be either health promoting or stress inducing—sometimes even hostile. If you seek longevity, surround yourself with people who are supportive and share positive values.

Finally, the larger cosmic influences such as seasons and atmospheric factors can have a profound impact on your health. For example, viruses and seasonal mood disorders are most common during the winter, and asthma and lung ailments peak during the fall. Understanding the rhythms of nature and the way changes impact your health, you can become proactive in adapting to environmental changes and thus preventing illness. This is the meaning of harmonizing with your environment.

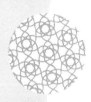

Greener Grass
May Not Be Better

Weed killers contain chemicals that are toxic to our nervous systems and have even been confirmed to cause cancer. If you want to live a long life, stop using chemical herbicides and artificial fertilizers on your lawns. Instead, fertilize with organic compost or manure, pull weeds regularly, and reseed areas that are overgrown. Do not cut the grass too short, as this will expose the root system and leave the grass vulnerable to disease. Also avoid lingering on the golf course too long, especially under a hot sun: extreme heat can strengthen herbicides' noxious effects.

Burn Clean
to Live Long

All efforts to protect our health are meaningless if an accident cuts life short. A few safety measures can significantly reduce these risks. Carbon monoxide poisoning kills more people than accidental chemical ingestion in the home. Because this combustion by-product is odorless, most people don't know when they are being exposed to it. Check the flames on your furnace, water heater, and stovetop. If you see a yellow or irregularly shaped flame, call the gas company immediately—you may be breathing carbon monoxide. Have a well-sealed door between your house and garage and keep it closed, especially when you start the car. Do not ever start up your car without opening your garage door first. Finally, be air-conscious: allow fresh air in from outside whenever possible.

Is Your
Workplace Fuming?

Energy-efficient standards dictate that modern houses and office buildings be kept tightly sealed to avoid temperature variations. This contributes to a condition known as "sick building syndrome," a nonspecific illness affecting a structure's occupants. Fumes emitted from carpeting, furniture, cleaning products, dry cleaning, insecticides, printers, and other products trigger responses from the immune system and eventually dull its efficiency, leading to premature aging. Circulate fresh air through your home or office by opening the windows early in the morning and late in the evening. Outdoor air is cleanest at these times of day.

Killing Bugs
Can Kill Your Cells

Pesticide sprays used in the home to kill ants, roaches, and other pests are made up of noxious chemicals that can shorten your life span. Researchers have found that children living in households that use pesticides have a much higher chance of developing childhood leukemia. Choose one of the many alternative, chemical-free pest controllers available at local health food stores.

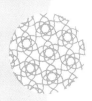

Check Your
Radon Reading

In outdoor surroundings, the radioactive gas called radon
is generally found in such low concentrations that it poses
no threat to human health. In enclosed buildings, however,
radon may build up to carcinogenic levels. Its presence
also varies by region, with areas rich in uranium deposits
showing especially high radon density. The gas causes an
estimated 20,000 cases of lung cancer each year. To find
out whether your house or office has high levels, you can
purchase a radon detector and send it to a laboratory for
analysis. The basic rules for minimizing radon exposure
are simple: seal all cracks in your basement floor, do not
sleep or spend prolonged periods of time in belowground
rooms, and keep your home and workplace well ventilated.

An Air
of Danger

Despite our best efforts to eat well, exercise, and keep
stress levels low, air pollution can shorten our lives. And
it's not just an outdoor problem. Particulate matter and
gases can contaminate the air we breathe in enclosed
quarters. Currently, the best air-purifying technology is
high-efficiency particulate air (HEPA) filtration, originally
developed for hospitals treating asthmatics. Its carbon
filters will sift out dust, pet dander, hair, pollen, mold,
mites, auto exhaust, and soot particles from printers and
copy machines. Some systems combine HEPA filtering
with a device that uses ultraviolet rays to kill airborne
bacteria, viruses, and fungi. Portable units can be pur-
chased at home appliance outlets. Remember to write
the date on the filter and change it at appropriate intervals.

You Can Run, But You
Can't Hide from Pollution

Running is an excellent form of cardiovascular exercise that can help city dwellers counteract those sedentary hours spent in the workplace. But runners in polluted cities breathe in more toxins than nonrunners, resulting in higher risks of lung disease. To minimize the amount of pollutants you breathe, jog early in the morning before rush hour, or run indoors on a treadmill in an atmosphere with fresh or filtered air.

Give Your
Food a Bath

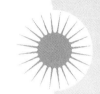

Go organic whenever you can to ensure that your food is free of pesticides and chemicals. When it's not possible to purchase organic items, be sure to wash and scrub your produce. Use a mixture of salt and hot water or a small amount of dishwashing liquid in hot water; fragile produce that cannot be scrubbed should be soaked in the solution. Rinse thoroughly. This process will remove external layers of pesticides, fungicides, and wax but unfortunately will not get rid of chemicals already absorbed from the soil during the growing period. For top quality, eat only produce grown on organic farms.

Peel Away
Pesticides

Unless your fruits and vegetables are organic, peeling off the outer layer may be the best way to reduce your exposure to harmful pesticides. Produce with the lowest amounts of pesticide residue are the hard-skinned fruits and vegetables like melons, squash, bananas, pineapples, corn, citrus, and avocados. Foods with the highest residue levels include some items that can be peeled—cucumbers, zucchini, peaches, plums—and some that are best eaten only when organic, such as grapes, cherries, celery, strawberries, and tomatoes. Of course, the downside to peeling is that you will lose some of the valuable nutrients found in the skins.

When You Clean Your Home,
Don't Pollute Your Body

Seeking longevity means protecting ourselves from products in the home that can compromise our health. Household cleansers containing bleach or chemicals are harmful when inhaled. Luckily, in the last decade natural cleaning products have come onto the market that are safe and do not pollute the environment. Better yet, some can even be made at home. For example, diluted vinegar is an effective cleanser for kitchen and bath tiles, toilet bowls, windows, mirrors, and carpets. The acetic acid in vinegar also inhibits bacteria and mildew. Just mix 1 cup of distilled white vinegar to 1 cup of water and use as you would any cleaning product. For scouring, scrub with baking soda instead of chlorinated powder.

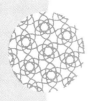

Detox
Your Oven

You may be dining on organic food prepared with the
utmost care . . . but has it been cooked on toxic surfaces?
Commercial oven and stovetop cleaners are poisonous.
When you're faced with a buildup of baked-on grease,
baking soda will do the job. Simply sprinkle it on, let it
sit for five minutes, then scour the surface with steel wool
or a scrubber. For more stubborn spots, mix dishwashing
liquid, borax, and warm water, spray the mixture on, and
let it sit for twenty minutes before scouring.

Let Nature
Fight Moths

There is nothing more aggravating than finding a moth hole in that new sweater you bought last winter. Don't resort to mothballs, though—they contain a benzene compound that causes cancer. Natural alternatives include cedar balls or panels and dried marigold, lavender, citronella, and pennyroyal, all available in herb shops. The safest option is to place your clothing in vacuum-sealed plastic bags for storage.

Unbleached Paper
for You and the Earth

Paper products are not naturally white. All white paper is bleached with chemicals that leave behind dense residues of dioxin, a known carcinogen. Such residues are found in coffee filters, paper towels, toilet paper, napkins, facial tissues, diapers, and lunch bags. When it enters the landfill as waste, dioxin also leaches into the soil, contaminating groundwater. Using unbleached paper products is good for both you and the environment.

Are Your Clean Clothes Toxic?

Traditional dry cleaning uses a chemical solvent, per-chloroethylene, to remove stains. Unfortunately, its chemical residue is toxic to humans. People often experience headaches, sinus congestion, shortness of breath, and dizziness from dry-cleaned clothing. Perchloroethylene also causes cancer in animals. To minimize your exposure, air out dry-cleaned items for at least twenty-four hours before placing them in a closet or drawer. To be safest of all, seek out dry cleaners that use organic, nonchemical cleaning methods.

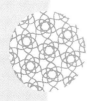

Furniture Doesn't
Have to Be New

That strong smell in new furniture, especially in items
made with pressboard and veneer, is largely due to the
formaldehyde used in adhesives. Formaldehyde can cause
strong allergic reactions and is toxic with long-term exposure. Shop for slightly used furniture, which will already
be adequately aired out. To avoid the chemical, use natural
wood furniture not made with pressboard or veneer.

Know Where You Are:
Locale and Longevity

No one wants to live near toxic dumps, nuclear power plants, or hazardous waste sites. But these are only the most obvious environmental dangers. With housing developments turning up everywhere, we may be unaware of toxins lingering from previous uses of a property. For example, living near land that was once a municipal dump could mean daily exposure to methane gas. Similarly, living downwind of a gas station or within one block of a dry cleaner exposes you to benzene and perchlorethylene fumes. Investigate a neighborhood's past and check out wind patterns before you decide to settle down. Preventing toxin exposure will pay off down the road.

Keep a Healthy
Electromagnetic Pulse

The human body's bioelectric system, like that of the Earth, has a natural pulsation rate. Both operate at an electromagnetic field (EMF) rate of 7.8 hertz. In household electrical wiring, however, the EMF rate is 60 hertz. Since most of the body's functions are regulated by EMF flow, the disparity between our bodies' pulse rate and that of our immediate surroundings can cause functional breakdown and imbalances. For example, children living near power distribution lines are twice as likely to develop cancer as those who do not. To minimize your exposure, keep a safe distance from sources of EMF. Stay four to six feet away from appliances such as microwaves, televisions, refrigerators, dimmer switches, electrical heaters, fluorescent lights, and electric clocks.

Grow Fresh
Air Indoors

Our homes should be our havens, places that nurture our health and soothe our spirits. These days, however, the synthetic materials found in buildings, furnishings, and electronic devices emit volatile organic chemicals (VOCs) into our home environments. These toxic gases include formaldehyde from plastic bags, benzene from wall coverings, and xylene from computer screens. Such indoor air pollutants aggravate allergies and fatigue; in severe cases they can lead to cancer and birth defects. Mother Nature to the rescue: plants are our best air purifiers. They produce oxygen and eliminate VOCs at the same time. Most effective are indoor palms, English ivy, ficuses, peace lilies, and chrysanthemums. So fill your home with houseplants and bring fresh air indoors!

Water,
Giver of Life

Since our bodies are composed of nearly 90 percent water, using pure water for drinking and bathing is essential to our health. The challenge, all over the world, is finding pollution-free sources of water. More than 700 pollutants, a number of them carcinogens, are regularly found in drinking water from municipal sources and rural wells. Research shows that water pollutant exposure through the skin is also a significant—and largely unrecognized—health threat. Filtered water is your safest bet. A wide-spectrum water filtration system can be pricey but will provide the highest-quality water for you and your family.

Make Your World
Less Plastic

Lightweight, durable, and versatile, plastic is a ubiquitous material in our modern conveniences. Many plastics, however, release vinyl chloride and other dangerous gases that can cause cancer, birth defects, and lung and liver disease. They also mimic estrogen in the body, leading to hormonal imbalance, especially in women. Besides the obvious plastics we can see—in our TVs, computers, telephones, coffeemakers, water bottles, and food containers—hidden plastics are found where you might least suspect them, in cosmetics, upholstery, carpeting, chewing gum, sanitary napkins, tissues, toilet paper, mattresses, building insulation, and polyester clothing. Cut your health risks by minimizing the use of plastic: use glass water bottles, wooden toys, paper products from recycled fiber, personal care products and cosmetics made with natural ingredients, and cotton or wool clothing, bedding, and mattresses.

Don't
Wear Toxins

The clothes we wear and our laundry customs can actually shorten our life span. Dyes containing benzidine, which is easily absorbed through the skin, are so highly carcinogenic that they are no longer used in the United States. However, the majority of clothes we buy today are imported, and many do contain such dyes. In addition, "no-iron" cotton fabrics are treated with formaldehyde resin, which releases fumes that can cause allergies, asthma, cough, headache, restless sleep, fatigue, and skin rash. When we clean our clothes with chlorinated laundry detergent and bleach, inhalation can irritate or damage the upper airway and lungs. Bottom line: wear naturally dyed cotton fabric, launder it in baking soda or natural detergent, and whiten with borax or nonchlorine bleach.

The High Price
of Artificial Beauty

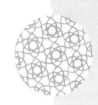

Ironically, when we use cosmetics we may be diminishing our actual well-being as we brush on that "healthy" glow. One of the biggest users of harmful chemicals is the cosmetics industry, and regulation is almost nonexistent. Examples are the formaldehyde in mascara, plastic resins in lipstick, asbestos-contaminated talc in eye shadow and blush, and chemical solvents in foundation makeup. All these substances are proven or suspected carcinogens. Natural alternatives found in health food stores use colored clays, vegetable oils, and other natural ingredients in place of chemicals.

Hair Care
That's Health Care

The human scalp is very porous and easily absorbs harmful chemicals. From hair coloring to shampoos and sprays, many commercial hair products are full of coal-tar dyes, ammonia, formaldehyde, plastic resins, and artificial fragrance that can cause everything from skin irritation to cancer or blindness. Natural alternatives to these chemicals are widely available in health food stores, or you can make your own. For natural hair dye, use strong black tea or coffee for a dark color or lemon juice for lightening. To shampoo, rub baking soda into your scalp and rinse—it does a better job than commercial shampoo, which can leave chemical residues on your hair. Orange water or honeyed water can be used as hair spray, and natural gelatin serves as gel. To preserve the gel, add enough vodka to make up about 25 percent of volume.

Get in Line— with Earth's Energy

Feng shui, or geomancy, is the study of energy meridians that crisscross the Earth and the practice of aligning with them. The planet is like a large, magnetized ball with positive and negative charges circulating up and down its longitudes, and the electromagnetic impact on its inhabitants is subtle yet profound. Arranging your surroundings in harmony with the earth's energy meridians will bring health, while violating this energy web can result in imbalance and illness. Whenever possible, your sleep position should be on a north-south longitude line. Some people find that once their sleep position is aligned, they have never slept better. Taking advantage of nature's gift is the ultimate purpose of feng shui.

Your Bedroom
Is Your Cocoon

Since you spend almost a third of your life sleeping, the
bedroom is the most important room in your home.
Ideally, your bedroom should be located away from the
entrance and from the street, in the quietest, least traf-
ficked area of the house. The decor should be minimalist,
not busy or distracting, in soothing colors like shades of
blue, green, or gray. Lighting should be dim, music tranquil. If you live in a noisy neighborhood, take soundproof-
ing measures to achieve a quiet atmosphere. The overall
feel should be cozy, safe, and cocoonlike.

Televisions and computers should not be placed in the
bedroom. These generate electromagnetic fields and
positive ions that can induce irritability and agitation.
You should not have plants in your bedroom, because at
night they give off carbon dioxide and deplete the oxygen
in the air you breathe. A relaxing ambiance in your bedroom will promote better rest, fundamental to good health
and long life.

The Energy Points of the Compass

The principle of feng shui is based on the ancient Taoist concept of energetic polarity. The terms *yin* and *yang* describe the opposite yet complementary energy states in the universe. A balance between the two polarities can help you stay in beneficial energy alignment and lead a healthy life. Yin embodies negative electrical charge and contractive energy, while yang is characterized by positive electrical charge and expansive energy states. The two yin directions are north (the negative pole) and west, the sunset direction. Yang is associated with south (the positive pole) and east, where the sun rises.

Activities in our lives can also be categorized as yin or yang. Sleeping, relaxation, reading, and bathing are yin activities, while exercise, cooking, engaging in hobbies, and studying are yang. Therefore, your bedroom and bathroom are more appropriately located in the northern and western parts of your home, and your office, kitchen, living room, and dining room should be in southern and eastern locations.

Flow Within,
Flow Without

Within our beings, energy and blood traverse hundreds
of miles of meridians and vessels. Disease, according
to Chinese medicine, is the result of stagnation and
blockage in either energy or blood. In our living and
working environments, too, energy can stagnate, creating disharmony and disrupting health. Arrange furniture
to promote natural movement throughout your home,
with special attention to corners, which tend to become
stagnation points and collect dust. Proper flow also
includes good airflow and cross-ventilation to clear
away stale indoor air.

Hug
the Ground

There are reasons why gravity keeps humans close to the
ground. For one thing, the higher you are from the surface
of the Earth, the less connected you are to the planet's
electromagnetic field (EMF). Our bodies' myriad functions
are regulated by our own EMF, which pulses to that of the
Earth. When this EMF synchronization is disrupted, disease
can result. Moreover, when you fly in a plane at 30,000 feet,
you are bombarded with a level of cosmic radiation similar
to one's radiation exposure in a chest x-ray. So whenever
possible, live and work no higher than four stories up, and
use air travel only when absolutely necessary.

Well-being Booster:
People

Just as we seek to create a healthy, positive, flowing environment in our bodies and our homes, building a human community with similar characteristics will benefit our lives. Being surrounded by family, friends, and associates who are loving, uplifting, and helpful to your well-being can add years to your life. A negative, depressing social environment, on the other hand, can sap the pleasures from life and rob you of the desire to go on. If you find yourself in the former situation, congratulations! Do everything you can to sustain it. If you're in negative surroundings, take whatever steps are necessary—only you can identify them for your particular case—to extricate yourself and develop a more life-affirming situation.

Danger
in Dampness

Dampness can be dangerous to your health. Weather conditions such as rain and high humidity encourage the growth of fungal mold that can be very hard to find or even invisible to the naked eye. In your home, improper construction such as poorly sealed windows, poor drainage in the landscaping, and belowground rooms can all contribute to mold infestation. Exposure to mold causes ill effects ranging from sinus ailments and headaches to serious problems such as intestinal conditions and liver damage. For this reason, it's important to repair water damage should it occur, ensure adequate sunlight exposure, and promote good air circulation throughout the house, especially in basements. "Bake" your home periodically by closing all doors and windows and turning up the heat to above 100° for a weekend while you are away.

Pots and Pans
Can Poison You

If you use copper or aluminum cookware, you may be
slowly poisoning yourself. The metals interact with heat
and food, leaching into your diet, and gradually accumulate in your body, sometimes to the point of toxicity. High
levels of aluminum, for example, have been linked to
memory loss, indigestion, headaches, and brain disorders
such as Alzheimer's disease. Toxic levels of copper can
impair the immune system and enable cancer cells to
proliferate. When scoured with abrasives, even stainless
steel cookware can release small amounts of toxic metals
like chromium and nickel. Nonstick pans contain Teflon,
a plastic that in recent years has been linked to immune
disorders and possible cancer conditions. If possible,
I suggest trading in your current pots and pans for cookware with porcelain enamel coating or made of cast iron,
glass, or lead-free terra-cotta clay.

Use Cell Phones
with Caution

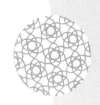

Convenient? You bet. Life-saving emergency devices? Sometimes. But cell phones have their downside. New evidence suggests that heavy use of cell phones may be bad for your health. Children under the age of eight should not use cell phones at all. Research indicates that mobile phone users are more prone to nonmalignant tumors in the ear and brain. Various studies suggest that cell phone use may cause changes to the DNA and cognitive functions and that cancer rates are higher near cell phone antenna stations. One potential remedy: the use of wired headsets coupled with magnetic beads. These inexpensive ferrite beads snap on to the wire near the earpiece end to reduce radio frequency radiation near the user's head.

Pride Goeth before a Fall—
Precaution Prevents Them!

Having fallen from a three-story rooftop, I can tell you first-hand that I am lucky to be alive. But most injuries and death from falling come not from dramatic incidents but from simply tripping over objects, slipping in the shower, or falling down stairs. You can take precautions to prevent falls: install devices such as motion detectors for lighting a dark hallway, use nonslip shower mats, and put handrails in the bathroom and along stairs. Get rid of clutter, tack down rugs, and rearrange furniture to create clear walking space throughout the house.

Poison Control
Begins at Home

Each year, poison control agencies receive more than
2 million calls because of human poisoning. The majority
of poisonings are due to drugs (illicit, prescription, and
over-the-counter), alcohol, carbon monoxide, and cleaning
agents. If you are interested in living a long and healthy
life, avoid drugs unless they are prescribed by your doctor,
and always ask the doctor for natural alternatives to drug
medication. Make sure that the drugs do not interact with
other medications, supplements, or botanicals you are
taking. Don't drink alcohol if you are on any medication,
and do not drink excessively at any time. Never sit in an
enclosed garage with your car running. Discard your
chemical cleaning supplies and replace them with natural,
nontoxic cleaning agents at home and at work.

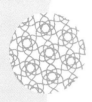

Too Close
a Shave

Nowadays we're all aware that some products contain toxic ingredients, and we're careful if we have to use them. For example, the carcinogenic chemicals called phenols found in laundry soap and household cleansers may not be an extreme threat—little or none remains on the clean clothing, and we can use gloves when handling cleansers. But when these chemicals are included in toothpaste and shaving cream, it's a different story. Both of these items are used near the mouth, so there's a higher risk of accidentally swallowing some. Phenol exposure via skin contact or fumes is always somewhat toxic, but ingesting phenols in even small amounts can cause respiratory failure and death. Your best bet is a good toothpaste from your health food store and a shaving cream made with natural almond or coconut oil. And while you're there, why not pick up some phenol-free kitchen cleanser and laundry soap?

Don't
Pine Away

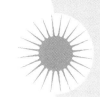

The wonderful scent of pine may evoke pleasant thoughts of winter holidays and crisp forest air. But when natural pine oil is concentrated and used in hair tonics, bath oils, disinfectants, deodorants, and other scented products, it calls for a healthy dose of caution. Pine oil can irritate mucous membranes in your nose and damage the skin. Never touch pine oil–scented bath oil until it is fully diluted in the bathwater. Above all, be careful not to accidentally ingest anything containing pine oil. This can lead to nausea, dizziness, chest pain, diarrhea, and headaches—even, in extreme cases, respiratory or kidney failure. Play it safe and enjoy pine in its natural form.

Bug Off
with Lemongrass

Commercial insect repellents will save you from mosquito bites, but many contain dangerous chemicals. Studies show that some ingredients can combine with other compounds, including prescription drugs in your system, to cause brain cell death and other neurotoxic reactions including seizures. A natural substance, lemongrass oil, also called Indian oil of verbena, is a better choice for keeping bugs at bay. Look for products in health food stores that use lemongrass oil to protect you from biting insects.

Jewelry . . .
to Die For?

One of the substances commonly found in jewelry cleaner
is cyanide—yes, the potent poison that can affect you via
fumes or skin contact. These small toxic exposures add up,
compromising our well-being over the long term, weakening us, and launching us into a premature old age. Luckily,
easy nontoxic replacements can be found right at home.
To clean gold, use toothpaste or baking soda and a soft
cloth. For silver, line a glass bowl with aluminum foil and
fill with three cups of hot water; add two tablespoons of
cream of tartar (available in the spice or baking section of
your supermarket) and allow it to dissolve. Soak silver jewelry in the solution for one hour, then rinse with plain water.

Flat
Is Good

The workplace can be a source of hidden dangers—even when the workplace is your home. If you use a computer in your home, you are exposed to electromagnetic radiation emanating from the cathode ray tube (CRT) of the monitor. CRTs operate at extremely high voltage (and thus high radiation levels), the larger ones using 35,000 volts or more. If you replace your CRT monitor with a flat screen type, you'll eliminate the risk completely. Flat screen monitors use a completely different technology; not only do they operate at much lower voltages (usually in the hundreds), they do not produce electromagnetic radiation at all. Oh yes, and as a side benefit, expect your utility bill to drop. You'll be using a lot less electricity to power your flat screen.

Toss Out That
Can Opener

Eating fresh food is a given in almost every medical tradition. In today's industrialized world, however, it is more important than ever, not just for the health benefits of locally grown produce but because of the dangers presented by the alternative. A substance used to line food cans, bisphenol A, is classed as an endocrine disruptor, a compound that can act like a hormone when it enters the human system. Scientists have found that exposure to such chemicals can contribute to prostate cancer, cystic ovaries, breast cancer, and endometriosis. To give your body the best chance for its maximum stint on the planet, boot canned foods out of the pantry.

CHAPTER 4: What You Do:
Exercise, Lifestyle, and Rejuvenation

The secret to longevity lies in action—engaging in the activities that make your body supple, your mind clear, and your spirit content. Centenarians' lifestyles are simple. They lead active lives and get plenty of rest. The centenarians I have known are dedicated lifelong learners and avid travelers. All of them seem to instinctively observe the natural rhythms within and outside themselves. Thus, by virtue of their good habits, they refrain from violating the natural order of the universe.

For most people, good habits must be cultivated. Brushing your teeth, for example, is a simple habit formed early on by parental reinforcement. If things were left up to children, we would all end up looking like our ancestors a few centuries ago, toothless at forty and headed for an early grave. Learning to form beneficial habits is critical to achieving health and longevity.

Chinese centenarians habitually practice tai chi and qigong, meditative exercises that have traditionally been associated with long life. They also take advantage of rejuvenation techniques the Chinese have known for thousands of years—like acupuncture, acupressure, and energy healing—that increase energy, promote health, and balance the body and the mind.

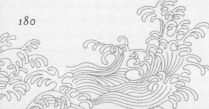

This chapter covers everything from the best time of day for exercise to rituals for a good night's sleep, from cognitive-enhancement exercises to breathing practices for eliminating toxins. These techniques, incorporated into a healthy lifestyle, seem to diminish the likelihood that your bad genes will be expressed. I have seen them work for countless patients and many centenarians with imperfect genetic histories.

Your choices about what you do can have a positive impact on your well-being, starting right now and for the rest of your life.

Long Walks
Beget Long Life

Every centenarian I have interviewed over the last twenty years walked for at least thirty minutes as a daily activity, and most walked more than an hour. It's no wonder they live to such an old age: studies have shown that walking can substantially reduce your risk of stroke and heart disease and raise levels of good cholesterol.

Time to Exercise:
Any Time!

We all know that exercise can prolong our lives, but many people say they simply don't have the time. In our busy routines, it may be difficult to find an hour or two every day to go to the gym or take a fitness class. I tell them that there are many opportunities to exercise throughout their day. My advice: take the stairs instead of the elevator. Park your car a few blocks away from where you're going. Cut the lawn with a manual mower. Sweep the floor with a broom instead of a vacuum. Wash dishes by hand rather than using a dishwasher. Walk to get your newspaper—don't have it delivered to your door. Every bit of physical activity adds up!

Pump Up
at Your Own Pace

Too often, I find patients coming in for injuries sustained from a new exercise program. This won't enhance your longevity! When starting any new exercise program, it's important to go at your own pace. Whether in a fitness class or working out with weights on your own, never force yourself or go beyond your comfort zone—when you start to feel any strain or pain, shortness of breath, dizziness, or sudden tiredness, stop! Know your limits. If you are not used to regular exercise, start with 10 minutes a day for a week, then go to 15 minutes a day the second week, 20 minutes the third. Continue to increase weekly, adding five-minute increments until you are comfortable exercising 45 to 60 minutes daily.

Make
Fitness Fun

Plenty of people engage in stop-and-start exercising—they begin an activity and then lose interest. But the key to benefiting from exercise is consistency. It's essential to find an activity you enjoy. This sounds like common sense, but I find many people wasting their money paying for a gym membership when they obviously dislike going there. Shop around until you find physical activities you like, whether dancing, rollerblading, jumping on a trampoline, golfing, or riding your bike. When you like what you do day after day, you'll have fun exercising.

Weights and Walking
for Stronger Bones

As people age, their bones become brittle and lose calcium. This condition, called osteoporosis, affects the majority of the world's population over seventy years of age. And no matter how much calcium and vitamin D supplements people take, without activities that exert weight on the bones, it will prove useless. We learned this when astronauts experienced weightlessness in space. Without gravity to put weight on their bones, they underwent much more rapid bone loss than they would have on Earth. This doesn't mean you have to become a weight lifter. Moderate weight-bearing exercises such as walking are sufficient to help restore calcium to the bones.

Aerobics Goes
to the Heart of Things

Whoever said aging is not for the faint of heart was right!
Your heart is a muscle that pumps the blood's nutrients
and oxygen throughout your body while transporting
waste products for elimination. A stronger heart means
increased tolerance for stress and strain. The best way to
strengthen the heart muscle is to increase your pulse rate
to 60 to 80 percent of your maximum heart rate (MHR)
when you exercise. Your MHR can be found by subtract-
ing your age from 220. For example, if you are 50, your
MHR is 170 beats per minute. Your optimal range of 60
to 80 percent would be calculated as 102 to 136 beats per
minute. Achieving this rate for 30 minutes a day, three
times a week, will help your heart to keep you going.

"Youth Hormone"
Factory: Your Body

Imagine a rush of rejuvenating growth hormones in your body without expensive injections or pills. Studies show that just doing squats and leg presses will boost your natural production of the "youth hormone" to several times the normal output. Increased growth hormone means increased muscle mass and strength, decreased fat deposits, more mental alertness, better sexual enjoyment, and elevated moods. Spike it up by weight training with fitness equipment, knee bends, push-ups, and rowing.

Bicycle for
Your Life Cycle

Besides being an excellent form of exercise, the act of pedaling a bicycle increases blood circulation to the lower body, especially the legs and feet, which helps to lower blood pressure. Bicycling for 60 minutes, three times a week, over a 10-week period dropped blood pressure an average of 13 points in a group of middle-aged people. Keeping blood pressure in range (below 130 systolic and 90 diastolic) is key to the prevention of strokes, heart disease, and kidney ailments.

Beat Diabetes
with Regular Exercise

Never lose hope in your longevity quest, even if you have a serious condition like diabetes. Sometimes the simplest things can improve your health picture substantially. Daily aerobic exercise can help reduce sugar in the bloodstream by causing the muscles to use up excess glucose (blood sugar), the hallmark of diabetes. Regular exercise can help patients with type I diabetes utilize their insulin more effectively. In others, aerobic exercise stimulates the pancreas to produce more insulin, virtually precluding type II diabetes.

How to Undo
an Ice Cream Sundae

The 300 calories you take in when you eat an ice cream sundae can be worked off by spending one continuous hour engaging in activities that are part of your daily life: mowing the lawn with a hand mower, gardening, sweeping, and ballroom dancing. So next time you decide to have that ice cream sundae or indulge in a couple of chocolate cookies, have some household chores lined up or go dancing afterwards. Personally, I'd skip the dessert instead.

Work Out
in the Water

Too many people find themselves disabled by worn hips and knees before they are old. This works against your longevity plans, because exercise is a crucial part of health maintenance. But many people suffering from joint pain can still reap the benefits of a workout thanks to water exercise. Besides swimming, water exercises such as water aerobics and "aqua jogging" using flotation devices have become popular in recent years. Water is the perfect cushion for joints and provides resistance for a good cardiovascular workout. Research shows that water exercise, though not considered weight bearing, still helps fight osteoporosis. Many health clubs now offer water exercise classes.

Play It Cool
in Summertime

During the hot season, keep a cool head: choose exercise activities that won't overheat your body. In summer your exercise routine should consist of swimming, ice-skating, working out in air-conditioned gyms, and practicing yoga and tai chi. Studies show that the risk of stroke is three times higher on warmer days than on colder ones. In fact, the peak months for stroke are June, July, and August. So in summertime make sure to drink plenty of water and exercise in a cool environment. Don't let the heat get to your head.

The Sun:
Friend and Foe

Many centenarians understand the power of the sun. They rise at dawn, and sundown is their bedtime. Sunlight, as we know, can be either helpful or destructive to our health, depending on our exposure level. The ultraviolet rays of the sun are a natural sterilizer, killing bacteria and fungus on the skin as well as promoting the production of vitamin D, a substance essential for bone health. It can also stimulate the immune system, raising the levels of natural killer cell activity. Too much sun exposure, however, can cause skin damage and more serious conditions such as skin cancer, heat stroke, dehydration, and suppressed immune function. To maximize benefit from the sun, limit direct exposure to thirty minutes or less daily, within two hours of sunrise or sunset.

Gardening Grows
Your Life Span

Centenarians around the world come from many different backgrounds and professions, but one of the most common hobbies among them is gardening. As exercise, gardening strengthens the muscles; as a discipline it requires patience and cultivates fortitude; and in the end it brings rewards and joy to its practitioners. Studies show that gardeners have a lower incidence of heart disease and osteoporosis than nongardeners.

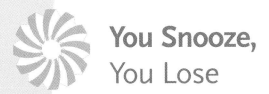

You Snooze,
You Lose

Staying active and exercising regularly are the foundations for living a long and healthy life. It's no surprise that caged animals have more health problems and a shorter life span than free-range animals. Research with humans confirms that as a rule, the more active you are, the longer you will live. In one study, the group that burned more than 3,500 calories a week lived the longest. Being lazy can actually shorten your life!

100 Million Tai Chi Practitioners Can't Be Wrong

Anyone who has seen images of China with masses of people slowly moving in choreographed, dancelike routines is familiar with the beautiful, health-giving art of tai chi. The fact that more than 100 million people practice tai chi around the world is a testament to its widely acknowledged benefits. Studies have concluded that practicing tai chi for thirty minutes, three times a week, for at least three months can slow bone loss in osteoporosis, lower blood pressure, lessen anxiety, improve sleep, increase functional mobility and balance, enhance circulation, and improve one's cholesterol profile. The best part is that tai chi is a gentle exercise that can be performed by anyone at any age. A majority of Chinese centenarians are practitioners. Tai chi classes can be found in community recreation centers and parks throughout the world.

Breathe
Away Toxins

Breathing, our first independent activity when we are born, is soon taken for granted as an automatic function. However, due to habits developed in response to illness, emotional trauma, and other experiences, many people do not breathe properly. It has been estimated that we eliminate only about 30 percent of the toxins in our bodies through defecation and urination—the rest are purged through the respiratory system. In other words, if you don't breathe correctly, you are accumulating toxins and wastes in your body. Practice deep, slow, rhythmic, diaphragmatic breathing daily, and you will reap the rewards of better energy, improved skin complexion, clearer mind, and elevated moods. Mind-body disciplines such as tai chi, yoga, qigong, and meditation all incorporate breath work into their routines.

Massage:
Not a Luxury Item

Most people enjoy massage for the healing effects and relaxation it affords. Yet many think of massage as a luxury. Its health benefits are worth every penny: a boost in the immune system, increased relaxation response, improved circulation of blood and lymph, relief from muscle pain and spasm, and many others. I consider it essential for good health and fitness. Of course, you can always learn to massage yourself or trade massages with a partner. Experiment with the many variations and styles, such as Swedish, acupressure, tuina, Thai, and shiatsu. With reflexology, simply rubbing your feet can produce an immediate sense of well-being.

Acupressure "Button" Turns on Your Immune System

A practice handed down over thousands of years, acupressure was first mentioned in writing in *The Yellow Emperor's Classic of Medicine*, the oldest medical book in the world. It involves warming an acupoint on the leg with the herb mugwort to stimulate the immune system. In this procedure, the practitioner rolls leaves of mugwort into a cigar shape, lights the roll, and holds the smoldering end near the acupoint. However, the same result can be achieved by applying firm, steady finger pressure. The point is found on both legs, about four finger-widths below the outside indentation of the knee next to the shin bone. Modern research in China confirms the efficacy of this treatment for improving immune function and preventing colds, flu, and infections. A healthy immune system will ward off cancer, infections, and degenerative illness.

Music to the Ears
Can Add on the Years

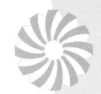

A traditional part of healing ceremonies and rituals throughout the world, music has a rich history of therapeutic use. In the last ten years, research has shown that slow, soothing music is generally good for one's health, while fast, stimulating music is not. Calming classical music not only enhances cognitive functions such as memory, concentration, and reasoning skills, but it also boosts the immune system, lowers blood pressure, relaxes muscle tension, regulates stress hormones, elevates mood, and increases endurance. Classical musicians, especially orchestra conductors, are among the longest-lived professionals. In studies, plants serenaded with soothing classical music lived longer on average than plants exposed to harsh, jarring music. If you're seeking longevity, that's worthy of note.

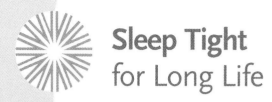

Sleep Tight
for Long Life

Mm-mm, a good, solid night of sleep. Nothing is more enjoyable or more healthful. Not only is sleep restorative to one's mind and vitality, it is also critical to the proper functioning of organs such as the liver, which performs most of its detoxification at night while you sleep. Sleep deprivation causes problems ranging from suppressed immunity, mood disorders, and digestive ailments to elevated cholesterol and blood pressure. Study subjects who stayed awake for seventy-two hours straight experienced an enormous drop in white blood cell production and activity—the measure of our immune function.

Longevity Prescription: Eight Hours of Z's

Research shows that chronic sleep deprivation can hasten the onset of memory loss and encourage diabetes and high blood pressure. Eastern medicine has long known that adequate nighttime sleep helps restore the yin (substance) that keeps the yang (function) in check. The conditions characterizing yin depletion and yang excess are exactly the symptoms that showed up in Western studies. The ideal sleep time recommended by ancient Chinese medical texts is eight hours. Average adults sleep eight hours and fifteen minutes when allowed to sleep as much as possible. Get at least seven to eight hours of deep, uninterrupted sleep to maintain good health and long life.

Sleep Rites
to Sleep Right

Our bodies run on biological rhythms and function best with consistent routines. To ensure restful sleep every night, form your own routines and rituals that help you go to sleep and stay asleep. Here are a few useful suggestions from my interviews with centenarians: hot baths, foot massage, journaling, meditation, aromatherapy, relaxing music, reading spiritual books, praying, and taking an evening stroll. These and other rituals help you calm your mind and feel peaceful within. Once you find an activity that works, be sure to practice it consistently to program your body for the sleep response.

Don't Quit
Your Day Job

Even if we are city dwellers, nature exerts a great influence
on our health and well-being in subtle yet powerful ways.
In Eastern medicine, it has long been believed that respect
for nature's cyclical changes brings health, and violation of
its rhythms leads to disease. Biochemical changes occur
when humans transgress the natural behavior patterns
associated with the division of night and day. Shift workers
on night duty and those with unpredictable working hours
have a 30 percent higher risk of heart attack than day
workers with set hours. Mice forced to live on a night-shift
schedule had a life span 11 percent shorter than normal.

Gymnastics
for the Brain

Having a few more senior moments lately? The dwindling memory, decreased concentration, and slowed response time associated with aging are largely caused by decreased blood flow to the brain and loss of brain cells. In addition to proper nutrition and exercise, mental fitness activities are imperative to prevent age-related cognitive decline. Read and learn new things, find new hobbies, do crossword puzzles, add up your bill in your head while shopping—all these can stimulate brain cell activities and in some cases even grow new brain pathways.

A Brush
with Longevity

A popular practice among centenarians is body brushing, using a dry brush with natural bristles to sweep the surface of the entire body. Besides eliminating dead skin cells and improving skin hygiene, body brushing can also increase small capillary circulation to the skin, boost skin immunity against infection, and promote vibrant skin tone. An alternative to brushing is body scrubbing: use a dry cloth or moist rag to vigorously scrub your body from head to toe.

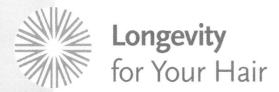

Longevity
for Your Hair

For many people, losing hair is more distressing than getting older. Hereditary factors obviously play a role in premature hair loss but for many others, hair loss can be reversed by natural methods. Start by eliminating hair care products containing harsh chemicals that can damage hair roots and strip vital nutrients from the follicles. Use only products with natural ingredients. Massage your scalp with your fingers or a hard-bristle hairbrush in a circular pattern. Apply the Chinese herb arborvita to stimulate follicles, improve blood flow, and strip away root-clogging oils. I have used this herb for my patients over the last twenty years with very good success. Of course, stress is a common cause of hair loss. Do your best to reduce it in your life.

Bend,
Don't Break

Bamboo is prized in Asia not only for the usefulness of its
sprouts as food, its inner stem as medicine, and its stalk
as construction material, but also for its cultural signifi-
cance as a symbol of flexibility. The supple plant is able to
survive even the most devastating storms. Our lives, too,
are filled with unexpected happenings, and those who are
successful at adapting to change have better health and
more fulfilling lives. Studies from China show that patients
possessing flexibility as a personality trait often recover
50 percent faster from illnesses than those who stubbornly
cling to their ways. Try not to become overly attached to a
specific outcome: stay on the course you have charted for
your life, but understand that when barriers present themselves you'll sometimes have to take a detour in order to
get back on track. Practice stretching, yoga, or tai chi:
being physically flexible can encourage the same trait in
your personality.

Warm Up, Cool Down,
When You Exercise

Many of my patients injure themselves engaging in even gentle disciplines like yoga and Pilates, because they don't take the time to properly warm up before exercise and cool down afterward. Our muscles get cold and stiff from even brief stints of sitting or lying down. I advise gentle stretching and warming your body with proper clothing or heat packs before you begin exercising. Many gyms and health clubs have saunas, an excellent way to warm up before an exercise session. Afterward, cool the muscles with a shower or use a cold pack, especially on areas where you feel muscle or joint pain.

Unhook Your Addictions
Holistically

Smoking, drinking, and drug addiction cause incalculable harm to the body and cost countless lives, not to mention the staggering financial tolls they entail. Drug-induced lung cancer, liver cirrhosis, and other diseases are all preventable and can be cured if addressed before they reach an advanced stage. The sooner you quit, the sooner your body will be able to start repairing the damages. Ask your doctor or specialist to recommend a holistic program that incorporates complementary and alternative medical disciplines in an integrated body-mind-spirit approach to drug detoxification.

For example, Chinese researchers have found that kudzu flower reduces craving and withdrawal from alcohol and other substances. Be sure your team is open to making such remedies part of the game plan. The good news is that it's never too late. Even with a long substance abuse history, once you stop, you can come to enjoy better health and well-being.

Ease Awake
to Ward Off Stroke

Strokes and heart attacks occur most commonly between six a.m. and noon. This is because when people arise from sleep and plunge into the activities of the day, their bodies experience a sudden and dramatic increase in blood pressure, temperature, and heart rate compared to their sleep state. This jolt taxes the system and creates strain on weak artery walls. Avoid literally jumping out of bed. It's better to gradually wake up with soft music, stretches, and self-massage before getting into the shower or driving.

The Chinese Taoists have passed down a morning ritual that eases the transition between sleep and wakefulness in a gently stimulating way. As soon as you wake up, massage your sensory organs: eyes, nose, lips, and ears. Gently tap and brush your scalp with your fingertips. Massage the rest of your body with a stroking action from your neck down to your shoulders, elbows, hands, chest and abdomen, hips, knees, and feet. Finally, massage your lower back by stroking with your palms. Inhale through your nose and exhale through your mouth three times to push out toxins. Then take three deep inhalations of fresh air to fill your cells with vital oxygen.

Take a Tip
from the Tortoise

Observe that in nature animals with a high metabolism
die early and those that burn energy more slowly can live
for many years. Take the example of the hummingbird: its
fast metabolism burns out the organism within two sum-
mers, whereas a giant tortoise can live past one hundred
years. Burning fuel to keep up a faster metabolic rate generates free radicals, which in turn damage cellular DNA and
produce a cascading chain of degeneration. Pace your daily
life so that activities are punctuated with rest and restora-
tion, avoid consuming stimulants, and reduce stress. Eat
appropriately for your circumstances: a light vegetarian diet
for those with sedentary habits, a higher-protein diet for a
physically taxing lifestyle. Don't "live fast and die young"—
instead be like the tortoise and get to the finish line!

Carotid Ultrasound
Keeps Strokes at Bay

Stroke is the third leading cause of death in the United States. More than $70 billion is spent each year to care for stroke patients. A blood test alone cannot accurately assess the risk of stroke, a catastrophic medical condition in which an artery bursts in the brain. Simple, inexpensive, and noninvasive ultrasound imaging of the carotid arteries, located on both sides of the neck, can better predict and prevent strokes. If you are over forty years of age, ask your doctor to order the test—it may save your life!

More Reasons
Not to Snore

Besides being annoying to your spouse, snoring can actually cause you to lose your life! Snoring puts the squeeze on the cardiovascular system by cutting oxygen to the blood, thus increasing blood pressure and leading to a buildup of harmful cholesterol. One study showed that snorers are twice as likely to develop heart disease and stroke as nonsnorers. To stop breathing through your mouth at night, sleep on your side, lose excess weight, and treat any sinus blockages you may have. If all else fails, see an ear, nose, and throat specialist. In some cases, excess tissues may be causing blockage of the airway, and surgery can help.

Take a Nap
to Kick a Heart Attack

One of the best ways to lower stress on your heart is to take a nap during the middle of the day. Chinese medicine has observed that, in the body's circadian rhythms, noontime is the peak hour for the heart. Therefore, Chinese doctors advise calming activities and rest at this time of day to maintain the health of the cardiovascular system. Researchers have found that men who napped at least thirty minutes a day were 30 percent less likely to develop heart disease than those who didn't nap. A siesta is a sign of wisdom, not laziness!

Get It off Your Chest: Lose Weight for a Healthier Heart

Nowadays, 61 percent of Americans are obese or overweight. That's no way to live longer! Obesity causes high blood pressure, which in turn makes your heart work harder. Most overweight people also have high cholesterol—another risk factor for heart disease. One study showed that when overweight people lost 10 percent of their body weight, they lowered their heart disease risk by 20 percent. So keep your weight down and give your heart a lift.

Is Longevity in
Your Job Description?

People in certain professions or positions tend to live
longer than average. For example, studies performed by
the life insurance industry show that symphony conductors and high-level company executives have lower-than-
average mortality rates. Chinese surveys have found doctors, artists, professors, and herb gatherers to enjoy a
lengthier average life span. On the other hand, some
industries are rife with injuries and stress that more often
cut your life short, including construction, manufacturing,
mining, transportation, agriculture, forestry, fishing, and
wholesale and retail sales. Notwithstanding the statistics,
it is important that the career you choose be meaningful
and enjoyable to you.

Stress-Busting
Flowers

Colorful flowers have a powerful influence on moods. A bouquet of flowers can conjure up love, uplift a patient's mood, and even help combat stress. A study showed that people who sat near a bouquet of colorful flowers were able to relax better during a five-minute typing assignment than those who sat near a foliage-only plant. Next time you want to relax or improve your mood, surround yourself with colorful flowers.

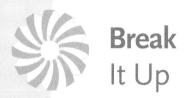

Break
It Up

Repetitive stress is not just for the office. As we age, many of the household tasks we once performed routinely cause fatigue, joint pain, and muscle ache. Some people believe that you should continue to perform them in the same fashion, under the assumption that the body needs to be challenged to maintain a constant state of strength. Chinese medicine, however, does not condone overextending one's limits. When you are vacuuming, for example, break up the job into small parts that do not tax your muscles for too long. Sweep half or a quarter of one room, then rest. Have tea or read a little, then resume the job. Use this method for any protracted work that tires your body. Yes, it makes the job longer—but it can do the same for your life!

Safe Car + Safe Driver = Journey to a Long Life

Car accidents account for nearly half of all accidental fatalities. The size of a car matters when it comes to safety. Insurance industry statistics found that the vehicle group with the lowest driver death rate was large luxury cars. The next lowest rate was in large minivans and station wagons. And pound for pound, across the vehicle types, cars almost always have lower death rates than pickups or SUVs. You'll want a safe car with features like airbags and seat belts, but it's equally important to drive cautiously, stay alert, and avoid strong emotional outbursts. Of course, one should never drive after drinking alcohol or taking medications that cause drowsiness.

Food Won't Sate
Emotional Hunger

Many people fall into the trap of eating to satisfy emotional hunger as opposed to physical hunger. Boredom, sorrow, pain, and emotional vacuums can trigger us to reach for comfort foods—which may actually give temporary content-ment by inducing the release of beta-endorphin in the brain. This reaction creates "food addicts" who use food like a drug to get temporary relief from emotional or physical pains. Food, unlike illicit drugs, may seem benign enough, but we have all witnessed the results of food abuse: obesity, diabetes, eating disorders, and depression, all of which can compromise longevity. Deal with your underlying unhappi-ness, and your food cravings and addictions will dissolve.

A Challenging Job
Can Ward Off Alzheimer's

Mentally challenging jobs may be stressful, but they force people to exercise their brains constructively. Coupled with effective stress management, a demanding job may be just what you need to keep your brain shipshape all the way into your old age. One study indicates that people who continually moved up to more mentally demanding jobs in the course of their careers may be less likely to develop Alzheimer's disease, which is currently incurable and always fatal.

Call a Slow
Moving Van

If you have lived in your home for some time and then change residence, by choice or circumstance, you may undergo some unexpected stresses. Here's how to avoid a health crisis: If possible, make your decision at least six months in advance of the actual move. Pack slowly, eliminating unnecessary items and enjoying the fond memories evoked by the ones you will keep. Say goodbye to each room, each corner, each window and door. Remind yourself that the good things that happened to you here are not located in this physical place; now they are memories that can never be taken away from you. If you can, visit your residence-to-be often during this time. Get accustomed to the lighting, odors, and feel of the place. Get to know a neighbor or two. If you haven't already done so, have the house or apartment checked for mold and mildew and be sure any problem is taken care of before the move. As soon as you move in, establish new morning and bedtime routines. Most of all, encourage positive thoughts about your long and happy future in your new home.

Chinese Methuselah's Longevity Secret

Peng Zu, the Chinese Methuselah who reputedly lived 800 years, is said to have invented *daoin*, a gentle stretching and meditative exercise that some consider to be the predecessor to yoga. One of the first moves of daoin is to take one of your heels and rub it against the sole of your other foot until you feel heat in the massaged foot, then reverse the feet and repeat with the other heel. Besides stimulating blood flow into the lower extremities, rubbing the bottoms of the feet activates an important acupuncture point for energy and vitality called Gushing Spring. Modern research shows that stimulating the point has a balancing action on the hormonal and nervous systems.

How to Guard
Your Energy Bank

In Chinese medicine, the abdomen is considered
the storehouse of the body's essence and energy.
You are well advised to carefully guard your energy
bank from potential robbers, which include the
weather, sexual excesses, dietary abuses, insufficient
sleep, and exhausting physical labor. Keeping the
abdomen warm and protected is believed to have
important health and longevity benefits. To replenish
your energy bank, regularly apply to your abdomen
a hot water bottle, abdominal wraps soaked in rejuvenating herbal solutions, or pouches containing
similar herbs.

Posture Maintains
Blood to the Brain

Poor posture leads to a drop in energy, affects your mood, and contributes to chronic back and neck pains. Slouching can make you look and feel older than you are. Additionally, slouching decreases your oxygen intake: when you compress the diaphragm and ribs, full respiration cannot take place and the blood flow to your brain and extremities is slowed. The Chinese remedy for poor posture is to pull your chin inward and pretend there is a string pulling straight upward from the top of your head.

Exercise Is a Promise
Not to Break (Your Bones)

Bone fractures are the main reason why people in the
United States end up in old age homes—and a frequent
reason they end up in cemeteries. Many times the broken
bones are due to falls. In addition to following the tips in
this book for strengthening bones through nutrition and
supplements, you can help prevent falls and fractures by
exercising the right muscles. Elderly people often lose
their balance due to weak ankles. Here's how to build up
the muscles that hold you upright: Sitting in a chair, hold
one leg straight out, parallel with the ground. Flex the top
of your foot as far back toward the shin as possible and
hold for 15 seconds. Repeat five times. Now rotate your
foot clockwise in as wide an arc as possible, slowly and
with isometric pressure, five times. Repeat in a counter-
clockwise direction. Do the whole set with your other foot.
Perform these exercises three or four times a week to
decrease your chance of a debilitating and possibly fatal fall.

Humming—A Sound
Health Habit

A good number of people affected by chronic fatigue have been found to have sinus disease, an impairment of normal gas exchange through the sinuses. Now, evidence suggests that humming along with the radio or crooning your favorite songs may help prevent or remedy sinus problems. Studies show that humming improves the output of nitric oxide, an indicator of effective sinus function. Also, humming is similar to the traditional practice of chanting, whereby sound waves elicit positive responses from your body and spirit. So, for better airflow and sound health, make a habit of humming on your way to and from work every day.

Whatever Does It for You, Do It Daily

Having a program of daily renewal is like sharpening your ax every day so that you may work with more effectiveness. While weekend spa treatments and yearly wellness retreats are refreshing and reinvigorating, their benefits are often short-lived unless you implement a sustainable daily program that reinforces your overall energy. Take time every day to do the one activity that always makes you feel good and have more energy, be it walking, doing tai chi, eating a bowl of fresh fruits and vegetables, soaking and massaging your feet, listening to classical music, or sitting and meditating. You will be rewarded with consistent performance.

Partner with Your Doctor for Proactive Health Maintenance

Many people leave their health care to their doctors instead of taking personal responsibility for their health objectives. While doctors are generally well trained to take care of disease, they are not trained to maintain your wellness. Make your yearly doctor visit a proactive one. Discuss your health goals with your doctor and have a written version included in your patient file. Ask for the results of your latest tests and compare them with prior ones. Check in with your doctor about all the medication, supplements, and herbs you are taking, and try to reduce or replace chemical agents with natural substitutes if possible. Educate and update your doctor about the latest discoveries or research on advances in longevity and healthy aging. Lastly, establish a cordial, respectful working relationship with your doctor.

A Body "Map"
Inside Your Mouth

In Chinese medicine, the tongue is seen as a "map" of the internal body. You can detect hidden problems early by inspecting your tongue for redness, cracks, or coating on specific areas. The very tip of the tongue corresponds to the heart. Crossing the tongue just behind this is a thin strip reflecting the lungs. The broad central portion corresponds to the spleen and stomach; thin strips along each side reflect the liver and gall bladder; and the back of the tongue is linked with the kidneys and bladder. Ask your doctor for further tests if you spot trouble in any of these areas.

The Eyes
Have It

You can learn to detect the early warning signs of disease by looking yourself straight in the eye. In Chinese medicine, swollen or reddish eyelids, for example, indicate digestive problems. Redness or irritation at the corners of the eyes may reflect stress to the heart. When the whites of the eyes are irritated and red, it means trouble in the respiratory and pulmonary systems. If the whites are yellow, this indicates jaundice, a sign of liver or gall bladder disorder, and requires immediately medical attention. Any changes within the iris may spell trouble for the liver, and dark circles under the eyes may mean hormonal imbalance, sinus allergies—or simply a need for sleep. To see inside yourself, inspect your eyes regularly.

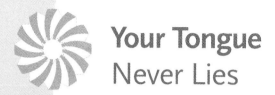

Your Tongue
Never Lies

Tongue diagnosis has a rich history in medical traditions worldwide. All ancient medicine employed tongue inspection to detect changes in the viscera or internal organs. The tongue is layered with immune cells that react quickly to intruders and is also filled with nerve cells and taste buds wired directly to the brain. It is fed by a complex network of blood vessels that changes the color of the tongue depending on the level of oxygen and nutrient delivery. The healthy tongue is moist and pink. A tongue that is red, cracked, or covered with a yellow coating signals an internal imbalance or illness. See your health care provider, preferably a doctor of Oriental medicine, if you notice these signs. For example, red prickles on the tip of your tongue may mean that you are under stress and have pressure or inflammation in your head or upper respiratory system. A thick coating on the back of your tongue may indicate toxins and waste buildup.

Say *Ha!*
for Healthy Organs

A common practice in China for health and longevity is to use healing sounds for organ health. Research has shown that certain sound waves induce relaxation and others stimulate bodily functions. The Six Healing Sounds are a simple technique that promotes the health of organ systems. All you have to do is utter each sound on exhalation for six breaths while visualizing the organ it is intended to stimulate. The sounds: "shoo" for the liver, "ha" for the heart, "hoo" for the stomach, "szi" for lungs, "foo" for the kidneys, and "shee" for the gall bladder.

Good Smells
for Good Mood

Smell has a powerful influence on our bodies and minds, research has shown. Stimulating olfactory nerves inside the nose activates the limbic system of your brain, which is associated with memory and moods. The use of plants with strong scents for healing and wellness, known as aromatherapy, is common among the world's medical traditions. Aromatherapy uses jasmine to treat depression, lavender for restless sleep, citrus to increase alertness, peppermint for poor digestion, rosemary for pain and muscle tightness, eucalyptus for sinus congestion, and patchouli for nausea. Essential oils of plants may be dabbed on your temples, at the back of the neck, or directly on acupressure points—or simply boil the herb in water and inhale the steam through your nose.

Spring: Cleanse with a Fast

Spring is a season of awakening. According to Chinese medicine, the liver and gall bladder are most active during spring. Our instinct to perform spring cleaning in our homes is reflected in the natural action of the liver to cleanse and detoxify the body. This is a good time to undertake liver-cleansing fasts, supervised by your natural health advisor. The 5,000-year-old *Yellow Emperor's Classic of Medicine* gives this advice: rise early and retire early, dress for cold mornings and evenings, stretch and exercise, and express your feelings freely. In this way you strengthen yourself against spring illnesses.

Summer:
Later to Bed

Summer is the season of tremendous growth and heat. Heat causes extreme expansion and promotes dehydration, which destabilizes the nervous system, lowers production of digestive juices, slows intestinal movement, and can lead to food poisoning and dysentery. Chinese medicine says the heart and small intestine are most active during the summer months. The Yellow Emperor's advice: early to rise and later to bed, rest during midday, prevent overheating during physical activities, drink plenty of fluids, add pungent flavors to the diet, refrain from anger, and maintain equanimity in order to prevent summer ills.

Autumn:
Time for Sour Flavors

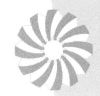

Autumn marks the turning point between the heat of summer and the cold of winter. The cooling weather ushers in the harvest and heralds the dying cycle in nature. The seasonal change also causes the respiratory system to constrict, leading to cough, asthma, bronchitis, and even pneumonia. Chinese medicine has always associated autumn with the lungs and large intestine. The Yellow Emperor advises early to bed and early to rise, practice breathing exercises, avoid pungent flavors but increase sour ones in the diet, drink fluids and eat soups, and remain calm and relaxed to avoid the diseases typical of autumn.

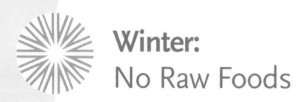

Winter:
No Raw Foods

The winter season is the sleep of nature. Days are short and nights are long. Humans long ago stopped hibernating like their ancestral cousins, but our bodies still experience the slowing of natural processes in winter. According to Chinese medicine, the winter season is linked to the kidneys, the adrenal glands, and the bladder. Toxins and carbon dioxide tend to accumulate due to inactivity; people are prone to colds, flu, poor circulation, and low vitality. Says the Yellow Emperor: sleep early and wait to let the sun bathe the house before rising from bed, dress warmly and engage in physical exercise, refrain from the cold and the raw in your diet, reduce salt to protect the kidneys but increase bitter flavors, be happy, and prevent the stirring of emotions. These are the ways to avoid the winter blues.

A Little Help
from Your Abs

In traditional Chinese teaching, digestive malfunction is said to account for up to 90 percent of all instances of disease. That is one reason the first section of this book, What We Eat, is such a lengthy one. Yet no matter how well we eat or which supplements we take, particles of undigested matter may adhere to the inner intestine, toxifying the system and preventing complete absorption of our food. One way to ward off this problem is to perform this simple "inner housecleaning" exercise once or twice a day, at least an hour after eating: With your knees slightly bent, lean forward and place your hands on your thighs just above the knee. Press down with your hands, exhale deeply, and draw your stomach in as tightly as possible at the same time. Holding your breath after full exhalation, use your abdominal muscles to push your belly in and out several times. Then stand up as you inhale. Repeat this three times. You will not notice an immediate effect, but over time every part of your body—from your skin to your brain to your sex organs—will benefit as all the nutrients in your food are absorbed and utilized.

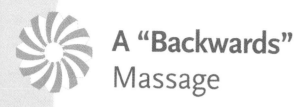

A "Backwards" Massage

Western medicine focuses so intensely on the blood that patients often know little about lymph, another vital bodily fluid. Lymph is a clearish liquid that drains impurities and cell waste for elimination. The fluid runs in the space between cells, but has no "pump" corresponding to the heart—its flow is dependent on the motions of your body and muscles throughout the day. When lymph stagnates it can produce edema (swelling) or allow toxins to accumulate. A special kind of massage is designed to get this system moving again. The practitioner applies gentle intermittent pressure to the lymph channels, working from the extremities toward the heart, the reverse of the direction in deep-tissue massage. Lymph massage is especially important for invalids, because they may stay motionless for long periods of time, but it is beneficial for everyone who seeks long life. Many types of massage therapists are also trained to work on the lymph system; be sure to ask your practitioner, spa, or massage clinic.

Your Hands
Can Help You Breathe

The science of reflexology allows us to treat ailments by stimulating certain points on the feet and hands that are linked with internal organs. Here's how reflexology can help keep your nasal passages clear during a sinus flareup: Hold your left hand in front of you, palm up. With your right hand, squeeze the base of your little finger and "walk" the thumb and forefinger up to the end of the finger, giving a little squeeze for each "step." Repeat for each of the other three fingers. For the thumb, start at the tip and move toward the base. Now do the same with the hands reversed. Easing congestion has obvious benefits for our longevity odds: we don't want to short the body of oxygen for even a brief time.

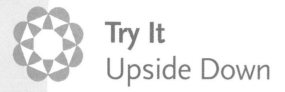

Try It
Upside Down

Like everything else in the physical universe, our bodies respond to gravity. As we age, we may think about this mostly when we fall down! But gravity acts on our internal organs, fluids, and skeletal structure as well. To keep them in top working order, it's best to occasionally reverse the pressure by turning our bodies upside down. Using a slant board with loops at the top for your ankles, position yourself at a gentle angle. Reversing pressure on the spine for as little as five minutes a day can allow compressed discs between the vertebrae to begin regeneration. Circulation to the brain is also improved (but be sure you don't stay so long that too much blood flows to the head). In addition, the pressure on organs is rearranged, and blood and lymph flow get a break from their routine.

Don't Let
the Bone Thieves In

A broken hip from osteoporosis can send you to an early grave. As you age, avoid the things that weaken the calcium in your bones. Some of the biggest offenders are nicotine, caffeine, and excessive alcohol, sugar, and salt. Caffeinated soft drinks are also very high in phosphorus, which actually removes calcium from your bones. Prescription drugs can do the same, including steroids and thyroid medication, so if you must take these, make sure your doctor closely monitors your bone health. Of course, weight-bearing exercise, exposure to a healthy amount of sun, and eating a diet rich in dark leafy greens, beans, and legumes can all help you prevent osteoporosis.

Keep Cool
on the Outside . . .

Experiencing extremes of temperature can endanger one's health and even one's life. To strengthen the body and make it more resistant to environmental temperature changes, I recommend taking cold showers. This constricts the blood vessels at the surface and extremities of your body, driving tremendous blood flow into the internal organs to increase oxygenation and transport waste away from these vital body parts. If you are not used to the practice, however, acclimate yourself gradually. Begin by scrubbing your body with cold towels. After a few days, run your shower or bathwater at a slightly cooler temperature than you are used to, and use less hot water each week until you can switch to a completely cold shower.

. . . and Warm
on the Inside

While cold is recommended for the surface of the body,
cold on the inside may be harmful. Most food and drink
should be consumed either at room temperature or close
to body temperature. Think about it: a glass of ice water is
about 35 degrees Fahrenheit, a differential of more than
60 degrees with the body's 98.6. Drinking cold beverages
constricts the blood vessels—just as cold does anywhere
in the body—decreasing blood supply to the stomach and
reducing the secretion of gastric juices, which can bring
about a decline in digestive function over time. It may also
weaken immune function in the digestive tract, leaving it
vulnerable to infection by the Helicobacter pylori bacteria,
the chief culprit in stomach ulcers. To keep your body in
top shape for the long haul, know how to run hot and cold.

Four Moves
to Checkmate Insomnia

Insomnia is a major contributor to the aging process and the breakdown of the immune system. The famous Taoist physician Ge Hong, who lived during the Han dynasty in the third century, promoted this set of exercises to treat and prevent insomnia. Chinese studies show that they dramatically improve the sleep quality of chronic insomniacs when performed nightly for two to four weeks.

In the first set, lie on your back with your knees bent. With your hands, pull your knees toward your chest and breathe naturally. Hold the position for one minute, then relax, straighten your legs, and rest your arms and hands at your sides. For set two, remain on your back, inhale, and stretch both arms upward above your head. As you exhale, bring your hands down and massage your body from your chest to your abdomen, then rest your hands at your sides. Repeat with every breath for about one minute.

The third set is also done lying on your back: Make fists with both hands and place them under your back as high as possible toward the shoulder blades, on either side of the spine. Take three complete breaths, then reposition your fists downward one notch and repeat, moving down-

ward every third breath until your fists are at waist level. Here, take five breaths, then position your fists on either side of the tailbone and take five more.

Lie face downward for the fourth set and place your hands under your abdomen. Slowly inhale, filling your abdomen and chest, and feel the energy permeate your whole body. Then slowly exhale and visualize negativity leaving your body. Pause after each exhalation and relax every muscle. Do this for one minute.

Sleep
Like a Deer

Ge Hong, a famous Taoist physician around 300 AD, firmly
believed in the possibility of physical immortality, and much
of his life was devoted to this quest. He recommended a
particular sleeping posture to follow the four anti-insomnia
exercises (page 248). After you have completed them, turn
partway over to sleep on your right side. This is called the
"deer sleep posture" because it resembles the position of
a deer asleep in the wild. Your right arm is bent at the
elbow, the palm facing up in front of your face; your left
arm rests with elbow on hip, hand dropped down in front
of your abdomen. The right leg is naturally straight, and
the left knee is bent, resting on the mattress in front of
your right thigh.

Early Detection
Prolongs Life Span

The Yellow Emperor's Classic of Medicine states that a superior physician treats disease before it occurs, while an inferior physician treats disease after it has manifested. To achieve longevity you must not only implement anti-aging measures but also prevent disease—this means detecting illness at its earliest stage. In addition to the annual physical exams you receive, both you and your health care provider should monitor your condition on a regular basis so that treatment can begin at the earliest possible opportunity. A simple home urine test to assess your level of free radicals is available from naturopathic centers and alternative doctors. It uses the by-products of free radical metabolism to detect these toxins in your urine, helping to determine the effectiveness of your anti-aging regimen.

Acuity Through
Acupressure

Cognitive decline such as loss of concentration and memory is a common symptom of aging. This self-help practice consists of stimulating two easy-to-find acupressure points on your neck at the base of the skull. Cross your hands behind you with the palms cradling the back of your head, your thumbs in the grooves on each side of your neck, and your index fingers crossing one another below the skull, just above the thumbs. Simply sit in a chair, lean your head back, and let it rest against the pressure of your thumbs and index fingers. Inhale through your nose and exhale through your mouth, slowly and deeply, and try to relax your whole body. Do this for three to five minutes. You'll increase blood flow to the brain and at the same time relax the neck muscles, which often tense up due to stress and constrict blood vessels in the area.

If You Fail to Plan, Plan on Failing Health

Health and longevity don't come about on their own—they need a little help. Most of us live in an environment rife with pollution, stress, and temptations to eat unhealthy food, and unless we act methodically to stem the tide of aging, we will be swept away. Be a planner. Write down specifically how you want to be and feel in weight, energy, mental acuity, and mood. What is your ideal for creativity, productivity, sexual potency? What symptoms of illness that you currently suffer would you like to overcome? Set realistic goals, then implement tips in this book to work toward fulfilling them. Once you reach a goal, revise it so you can continue to improve and progress. There is no limit to how healthy, how well, how energized, you can feel. Plan on feeling your best.

CHAPTER 5: Who You Are:

Genetics, Relationships, Love, Sexuality, and Faith

Overindulgence of the five emotions damages the energy that protects and nourishes the five organ systems. When the energy is injured, the body is vulnerable to attacks . . . yin and yang become divergent, organs are malnourished, disease and even death may ensue shortly thereafter.

The Yellow Emperor's Classic of Medicine

To accomplish any goal in the distant future, we must start from the here and now. If health and longevity are your aims, then you must understand what has made you who you are today. To start with, you are the physical and spiritual fusion of the ancestors whose genes you carry. Knowing your family medical history is a starting point in the pursuit of knowing yourself.

Human beings are complex social creatures that evolve and adapt to external changes. Your relationship with the people in your life—your parents, siblings, grandparents, cousins, children, friends, coworkers, and neighbors—all help to shape your health picture and your emotional experience of life. It has been said that it takes a village to raise a child. Well, in like manner, it takes a village to make a centenarian! Building a community of people around you to help you achieve your goal is fundamental.

254

We all have a constitutional archetype. Do you run hot and hyped up, or are you cool and measured? In addition, we have the responsibility to manage our own tendencies. When you mismanage your emotions, you are out of control. The result is stress—the underlying cause of up to 80 percent of all chronic diseases. Conversely, a deep belly laugh can give your immune system a huge boost!

It's not surprising that happily married couples live longer and healthier lives on average than single, unmarried persons. Besides the emotional security and fulfillment that comes from a committed marriage, partners reap the regenerative benefits of sexual intimacy. Studies show that sexually active seniors are the happiest men and women in any age group.

So what's love got to do with it? Love is a powerful force of nature. In order to harness its energy, you must first cultivate love of self. Only then will you be able to love and be loved. Romantic love can be a double-edged sword, however, sustaining those who have a mate but cutting down those who lose one. It is commonly observed that among senior couples, when one person dies, the other quickly follows. Universal love, on the other hand—or the closest human feeling to it, maternal love—frees you from the anguish of separation and desire. It unites you with the source of the essence that is the same in every animate and inanimate thing.

Your spirituality and personal faith are the hidden elixir in your life. Cultivating yourself spiritually, strengthening your connection to the universal divine, or God, no matter what your spiritual or religious faith, will bring you inner peace and the ability to cope with life's troubles. Study spiritual works, apply your learnings to improve your life, practice prayer and meditation, and express universal love through service to others, and your evolution will not only enlighten you but add years to your life.

This chapter offers tips for building harmonious relationships, meditation techniques for connecting with the divine, and sexual practices for health and wellness. Use them well and you will be on the path to a happy, healthy, and spiritually fulfilled life.

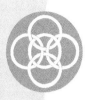

To See the Future,
Look to the Past

Heart disease, stroke, diabetes, and cancer, the deadliest diseases in the industrialized world, are often genetically inherited. To help prevent the development of genetically susceptible diseases, it's important to know about your family's medical history. Starting with your parents and grandparents on both sides, then your first cousins, learn each relative's health picture and, for those who have passed away, the cause of death and length of life. In the last fifty years, the human life span has increased dramatically, mainly due to early detection and treatment of disease, so do not fear if many of your ancestors died prematurely of a medical condition—chances are there is a modern cure. If your ancestors lived long lives, consider yourself lucky, but do not become complacent. Instead, do everything you can to ensure that you give your favorable genetic heritage the best possible chance to express itself in you.

Spiritual Faith
Can Conquer Illness

Many centenarians around the world come from poor, disadvantaged backgrounds. Others have experienced personal struggles, tragedies, or illnesses in their lives. However, they all share a common characteristic—strong spiritual faith. Faith is a belief in a higher power, universal order, or force behind creation that some call God. Faith allows one to find peace within, to accept what is, and to reconcile the difference between one's expectation and reality. I have personally seen patients overcome terminal illness due to spiritual faith. As one patient who overcame liver cancer said, "I have given my problems to God, and I've lived to be 100!"

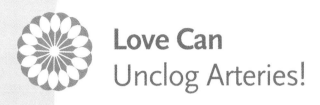

Love Can
Unclog Arteries!

Loving unconditionally and accepting love from others
makes your life not only meaningful but healthy. Researchers
have found that tender, loving care reduced atherosclerosis
and risk of heart attack in rabbits fed with high amounts of
cholesterol. Even watching movies about love or subjects
that inspire altruism has been shown to increase levels of
immunoglobulin-IGA—the first line of defense against cold
and flu viruses.

Rx for Aging:
An Active Sex Life

The majority of seniors experience a precipitous drop in the frequency of sexual activity as they age. As a result, they miss out on nature's secret fountain of youth: healthy sexual activity. It can raise the levels of substances that lengthen your life span—such as endorphins, growth hormone, and DHEA—and lower those that can shorten it, like the stress hormones adrenaline and cortisol. And sexually active seniors are simply happier. Fulfilling sexuality not only improves the quality but the quantity of your years!

Three Keys
to Healthy Sexuality

Chinese medicine has long recognized the power of sexuality
for health, longevity, and spirituality. Appropriateness and
naturalness are the hallmark of healthy sexuality. Accordingly,
there are three principles of healthy sexuality. The first principle: be aware of your needs and make sure to communicate
them. Do not force the act if it does not feel natural, if your
energy is low, or if conditions are not safe and conducive.
The second principle: be in tune. Follow the seasons and
observe that in nature animals tend to be more sexually
active during spring and summer and less so during autumn
and winter. Frequency of sex also depends on your state of
health. The third principle: Be considerate. It is equally
important to gauge your partner's mood, energy, and needs
so that you may respect and accommodate them. Achieving
satisfaction for both partners is the first step toward reaping
the benefits of sexuality.

Taoist Sexual Practice
Invigorates Body and Soul

As we know instinctively, sexuality that promotes health, longevity, and spirituality is more than just the act of copulation. The ancients believed in the productive transformation of energy during sexual activities. They developed a discipline using techniques of sexual practice with roots in Taoist tradition. Indeed, as Chinese research suggests, correct sexual practices yield immense physical and emotional benefits to participants ranging from elevated mood, relaxation, and increased circulation to balanced hormonal production and improved vigor. In contrast, poorly performed sex acts yielded little or no benefit and may even be harmful, possibly subjecting the participants to emotional or physical trauma. Learn the sexual techniques of tantra, from the yoga tradition, and fang-chung, from Taoist teachings, and sex can become part of your longevity plan.

Loving Family,
Long Life

Centenarians are beloved by their family members, and studies show that people with happy family lives tend to have less illness and a longer life span. A good familial relationship does not necessarily come automatically, but it is worth the personal effort to build and maintain one. Investing in your relationships can pay dividends in a life rich in love, respect, and a sense of belonging. Fill your family with happiness based on trust, mutual help, love, peace, listening, humility, honesty, justice, and sharing.

Be a
Good Neighbor

Spiritual literature throughout the world has promoted
one theme throughout the ages: love your neighbor,
and treat others as you wish to be treated. Neighbors
are an important part of your supportive community. I
have heard stories of patients' lives being dramatically
changed by neighbors who came to their aid in times
of need. Neighbors are like extended family, providing
friendship and community to help you avert loneliness
and isolation, promoting a longer, happier life.

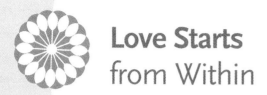

Love Starts
from Within

Love is the most powerful emotion you will ever experience, and studies show that while you are feeling it, endorphins and immune cells are produced in great number. How can you nurture this life-lengthening emotion? As a child, you learn to love your parents, your pets, your siblings. As an adult, you come to love your spouse, your children, and your friends. But have you learned to love yourself? To truly love others, you must first understand and experience love of self. Only then will you know how to love and appreciate those around you. Every day, do at least one thing that promotes love of self: engage in an activity that makes you happy, repeat affirmations of positive self-imagery, or even write letters to yourself as if to a new lover!

Universal Love Unites
You with the Eternal

God is nature. The expression of God in human nature is
universal love. It is within us, not outside of or separate
from us. Universal love is the capacity to embrace all in
the universe, from the smallest ant to the unfathomable
sky, the beautiful and the ugly, the good and the bad.
Universal love can disarm all prejudices, dissolve all differences, and bring the mind back to one core awareness—
that everything comes from the same source. By realizing
and practicing universal love, you learn to accept yourself
and your life and become part of the larger life, which is
the eternal universal divinity. How can we do so? Practice
gratefulness by appreciating the sources and people that
make it possible for you to have what you have, be it food,
clothing, shelter, job, education, or a relationship. Practice
kindness by looking for opportunities to make someone
feel happy: sweep the sidewalk in front of your neighbor's
house, give up your seat on a bus to an elderly person,
bring food to the homeless. Once you begin, you will find
many pathways to universal love.

Be Good to Others
to Be Good to Yourself

Compassion, kindness, and willingness to serve others are natural virtues in human nature. These traits dissolve your ego, which keeps you separated from others. Compassionate people understand others, have empathy for them, and are less likely to become angry, which can lead to stress and hypertension. Cultivating compassion is the first step to experiencing love of humanity. From compassion emerges kindness, which manifests in the selfless action of service to others. Kindness generates goodwill and dispels hatred and competition, feelings that diminish both quality and length of life. Researchers have discovered that selfless, altruistic service not only promotes love, peace, and understanding, but also produces natural killer cells that protect you from infections.

Travel Light:
Forgive and Forget

My father taught me this: "Forgiveness is the power that
enlivens relationships. Forgiveness keeps life moving forward, creates love and harmony, and makes you spiritually
strong." Once you forgive, you should also forget. The
benefit of this letting-go is that you no longer carry your
unpleasant experiences with you on life's journey. Many
people bear the baggage of the past throughout their
lives, and the more they have, the sicker they may be. One
unique characteristic of centenarians is that they are quick
to forgive and forget. They swiftly move on from negative
experiences and celebrate the positive ones in their lives.
By exercising your powers to forgive and forget, you will
deepen your relationships, enriching and prolonging your
life in the process.

To Be
and to Do

To be or not to be? To do or not to do? These conundrums
are forever troubling us. Perhaps not as an answer, but
more or less as a guide, ponder what a Chinese sage once
said: "By the light of the virtue of balance, you will see the
appropriate course of action, the appropriate way of life, and
the appropriate role to play. You will always courageously
and fearlessly steer the right course." In other words, from
a place of balance you will find a natural appropriateness
working through you to restore righteousness in your life.
This wisdom will keep you on the path to longevity.

The Alchemy of Tolerance:
Negative Becomes Positive

You can expand your emotional elasticity by cultivating tolerance. Greater emotional flexibility increases your ability to flow with the ups and downs of life. You are less affected by disappointments and traumas. Tolerance enables you to make your sufferings seem small and your blessings seem big. Nurturing tolerance can help you transform potentially stressful negative situations in your life into positive situations with a beneficial outcome.

Tool against Temptation: Self-Respect

Self-discipline is an essential virtue for achieving success in any endeavor. If living a long, happy, and healthy life is your goal, then governing impulses and resisting temptations are critical to your success. Self-discipline comes from self-respect. Respect the wondrous opportunity of being alive, and respect your body as the temple of universal divinity. Your true nature will help you control urges for instant gratification and stop you from taking the wrong course.

Simple Living, Self-Reliance: The Mark of All Centenarians

In studying centenarians over the last twenty years, I have discovered the power of self-reliance. They all led simple, clean lives with little or no extravagance. Fiercely frugal, obtaining the most from the least amount of resources, they seemed to take pride in self-reliance. Even those well past the age of 100 were still performing their own daily chores. A Chinese sage once said, "Modesty brings contentment, and all things grow well in the absence of clutter and complexity." Conserve your resources, and do not let others do what you are capable of doing for yourself.

Snuggle, Cuddle, Hug— It's Good for You

Throughout the ages, hands-on healing has been recognized as a powerful technique. Researchers have long observed that orphaned babies stop growing and even die from the lack of touch and love. Similarly, unconscious patients who are regularly touched recover faster than those who do not receive touch. Human touch elicits elevated production of endorphins, growth hormone, and DHEA, all of which lengthen your life span, and touch lowers the levels of stress hormones that can shorten it. Hugs can achieve the same thing. Grandparents cuddling their grandchildren, friends hugging one another, and spouses snuggling up to each other all achieve this beneficial effect.

Stress Can Be an "Inside Job"

Stress is usually caused by an external stimulus, but our responses play a big role in how it will affect us. Consider the study of two groups of mice in which one group was exposed to a live cat outside their cages, and the other was exposed to an identical toy cat. The live cat group of mice developed more diseases and lived only a third as long as the toy cat group. The mice apparently figured out that there was no real danger from the toy cat and eventually simply ignored it. By reframing our perspective on stressful situations, we can often see that the danger is largely an illusion. When we moderate our reactions to potential stressors, we too can neutralize negative situations.

Meditate, Don't Medicate

For thousands of years meditation has been practiced in the East as a tool for inner peace and spirituality. There are as many meditation techniques as there are traditions. Mostly, the discipline involves practices of breathing and visualization techniques. The effects of regular meditation have been well documented by studies. Its benefits include lowered blood pressure, less heart disease, decreased chronic pain, and increased mental clarity. Often, it only requires fifteen minutes of practice daily to enjoy the health benefits of meditation. There are plenty of meditation courses on tape or CD that you can purchase in bookstores, or look to your local yoga or tai chi studio for classes on meditation. Start meditating today and feel your tension melt away.

Be Like a Two-Year-Old— Just Say No!

The biggest stressor for many people is their attempt to please everyone. We feel the most calm when we are in control. When we are overcommitted, we feel overwhelmed and out of control—and therefore stressed. There is power in the word *no*, and we should relearn it and use it. When we are able to acknowledge our limitations and our need for peace by saying no to additional burdens, we reclaim control of our lives and reduce stress. Remember how powerful it felt when you uttered the word *no* when you were two?

Prescription for Longevity:
A Happy Marriage

Research has confirmed that happily married couples live on average four years longer than single people. The emotional and psychological fulfillment derived from a satisfying long-term relationship helps individuals to weather life's challenges and difficulties without the worst depredations of stress. Psychologists also attribute the increased life span to the sense of interconnectedness to another human being. According to one study, nearly 100 percent of male centenarians are married or have only recently been widowed.

Qigong
to Exhale Stress

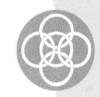

Besides detoxifying the body, specific breathing techniques can relax, revitalize, and regenerate your being. Qigong is one such breathing technique from China. In this practice, you must become mindful of every breath you take: monitor the speed, temperament, and depth of inhalation and exhalation. The goal is to slow down, smooth out, and deepen each breath. With every exhalation, utter the word *calm* in your mind and breathe out the tension from a part of your body, starting from the top of your head and working your way down through each part of your body until you get to your feet. Release the remaining tension through your toes and the bottoms of your feet.

Speak Your Mind
for Peace of Heart

Acknowledging our feelings is one of the most powerful ways to neutralize negative emotions. When we do so, we ward off the floods of damaging stress hormones such emotions produce in our bodies, potentially shortening our lives. Let people know when you feel unhappy, disappointed, or hurt about something. Once the feeling has been acknowledged by you—not necessarily by others—it tends to dissipate and is less likely to trouble you. If you hold your feelings inside, you are apt to explode at some minor incident, potentially causing still more harm to your health. Own up to what is in your heart and make peace with it forever!

Take a
Mental Dump Daily

If you don't have a bowel movement for several days, you're not only constipated, you're filled with wastes and toxins that can damage your health. The same thing happens with our minds. Negative thoughts, feelings, and images can linger and become "toxic," affecting our thought patterns and behaviors subconsciously. To quell this "mental constipation," write in a journal at the end of the day to unload all the negativity you have experienced. Writing it out allows you to reflect, understand a situation, and observe your feelings. For the ultimate elimination, rip out the journal pages and burn them. You will feel clearer and lighter in your being.

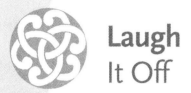

Laugh
It Off

The late Norman Cousins helped pioneer "laugh therapy" as well as the new medical discipline of psychoneuroimmunology—the study of the mind's impact on the body's immune functions. He and other researchers discovered that laughter and joy boosted immune functions, particularly production of the natural killer cells that defend the body against infections and cancer. Laughter also brought about increased endorphin release in the brain. There is no question that joyful people live longer, healthier lives. Read the comic strips or watch your favorite comedy show and laugh all the way to the longevity bank!

Cut Clutter,
Slash Stress

Simplify your life by cutting out the unnecessary items
and activities that collectively consume a large chunk of
your energy—resources that can be devoted to your health
and wellness. The fast-changing world we live in lures us
to acquire more and more objects. The more we consume,
the more we become enslaved by our belongings. Look
around your house, find things you haven't used in the
last three months, and give them to charity. Clutter makes
you disorganized, adding to your stress level. Streamline
your surroundings to stay calm and in control.

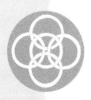

Cancer Breeds
in Repression and Stress

Nowhere is stress more directly linked to the development of a disease than in cancer. Patients with cancer are more likely than the general population to have suffered severe personal loss at an early age or to have experienced chronic depression with strong, persistent feelings of helplessness and hopelessness. People who have experienced prolonged stress and those with type C personalities—characterized by a strong tendency to deny and repress their own feelings—are much more prone to developing cancers. Many more recent studies have confirmed the effect of emotional stress on the body. Neuroendocrinology is one of the new fields to emerge from these studies on the connections between the mind and emotions on the autonomic, immune, and endocrine systems.

What Color Is Your Spleen?

This is a simple meditation practice that can help you energize your internal organs. Five Clouds meditation involves visualizing the colors associated with each of the five organ systems that keep us alive. It is an ancient meditation practice found in the *The Yellow Emperor's Classic of Medicine*. The five elemental colors corresponding to the five organ systems are green for the liver, red for the heart, yellow for the spleen, white for the lungs, and blue for the kidneys. Start by imagining a gathering cloud of the corresponding color enveloping the organ, in the order given. Take about two to five minutes for each organ system. Once you have completed all five color clouds, expand them all so that the five colors intermix and ultimately become a rainbow.

Your Early Warning System:
Awareness Meditation

Becoming aware of your body's natural states can help
you detect subtle changes in your health. This awareness
meditation is a powerful, easy practice that can be done
anywhere and anytime. For one minute, close your eyes
and be attentive to your breath. Is your breath fast or slow,
shallow or deep, short or long? Can you feel your lungs
and abdomen expand and contract as you breathe? Next,
for one minute, extend that awareness to your entire body.
Is there discomfort or pain anywhere? Can you feel your
digestion working? Is there movement within your
abdomen? How are you sitting or lying? Can you feel the
flow of energy and blood throughout your body? Finally,
for one minute, expand that awareness to your outside
environment. Experience the lighting conditions, temperature, subtle sounds, odor, and people nearby. What is your
reaction to them? Record your observations in a notebook
and review regularly for any subtle changes that may
require attention.

Happy Heart,
Healthy Heart

According to Eastern medicine, joy is the emotion associated with the heart. It has long been observed that happy-go-lucky people are less likely to develop heart disease, and science confirms this. One study showed that one in five patients with coronary heart disease comes from the population of the severely depressed. Cancer researchers found that pleasurable emotions increased levels of natural killer immune cells. Take steps to "practice" joy in your daily life, and it will expand naturally. Let joy fill your heart, and your heart will gladden your health.

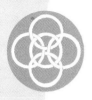

Managing Anxiety in a Crisis

People often unknowingly aggravate stress with their anxiety during a crisis period, leading to more stress hormone production and further damage to their health. To reduce anxiety, talk about your fears to friends, family, coworkers, mentors, or when necessary a psychotherapist. Eliminate stimulants such as caffeine from your diet— and from your medication, which may include caffeine and ephedrine compounds. Write down the worst-case scenario to your fears and then burn it, allowing it to leave your life.

Your Health
Is Your Business

To live healthy and long, the first thing you must do is to take responsibility for yourself and your life. Independence is a common quality among centenarians, many of whom see to their own daily affairs until the very end. If you depend on doctors to keep you well, you will surely be disappointed. Learn about your own health and implement steps to improve and maintain it. This means controlling unhealthy impulses for instant gratification, "owning" your disease so that you can change it, and exercising forgiveness and acceptance of yourself so that you can evolve. Taking responsibility for yourself also gives you the power to change—from illness to wellness, sadness to happiness, conflict to peace.

Invocation for Health and Longevity

The power of intention can create physical responses, as proven by biofeedback and mind-body research. It can also elicit energetic response from the divine universe. Traditionally, an invocation is a verse recited aloud or silently with mental and spiritual intentness on a beneficial outcome. From the Taoist longevity tradition, I will share with you this Invocation for Health and Longevity from the *Workbook for Spiritual Development* by Hua-Ching Ni:

I am strong; the sky is clear. I am strong; the earth is solid. I am strong; humans are at peace with one another. My life is supported by the harmonious spheres of body, mind, and spirit within my being. All of my spiritual elements return to me. All of my spiritual guardians accompany me. The yin and yang of my being are well integrated. My life is firmly rooted. As I follow the path of revitalization, my mind and emotions become wholesome and active. The goddess of my heart nourishes my life abundantly. Internal energy balances my spiritual growth, and all obstacles dissolve before me. My natural healing power contributes to a long and happy life, so that my virtuous fulfillment in the world can be accomplished. By following the subtle law and integral way of life, I draw ever closer to the divine source of health and longevity.

"Effortless Being" Means Longer Life

The renowned Chinese sage Lao Tzu promoted a concept and practice called *wu wei*, which means effortless being and doing. *Effortless being* means to be natural, unforced, and adaptive. *Effortless doing* means not applying undue energy or force to anything. Most people struggle unnecessarily through life, battering down walls instead of finding the doorway. Many exhaust their energy digging in dry, hard soil instead of softening it with water beforehand. Keep these metaphors in mind and translate them to daily life. For example, in relationship conflicts, the more you try to control the outcome, the more the fight escalates. Allow anger to settle on both sides first—let the fire burn out completely, rather than getting singed while rummaging through the ruins. If you practice wu wei in your life, you will be rewarded with increased joy, flow, health, and longevity.

There Are No
Greedy Centenarians

When controlled by their desires, human beings soon become worn out and broken in health. Greed for food, sex, money, and power becomes an addiction and an obsession, even though the inclination to seek them may have originated in a natural survival instinct. The wisdom you use in fulfilling your basic instinctual desires will determine your success in achieving self-preservation. Successful centenarians know that the key to long life and health is having control over their desires, not being controlled by them.

Your Face Tells
Your Elemental Body Type

In Chinese medicine, determining an individual's body type allows the doctor to prescribe advice corresponding to the patient's individual constitution. The easiest way to ascertain your body type is by the shape of your face. (Even though facial contours may change a bit as weight fluctuates and as we age, the basic shape remains fixed.) For example, a rectangular face shape represents the "wood" body type. The other four pairs are: square face shape, "metal" body type; inverted triangle, "fire" type; inverted trapezoid, "earth" type; oval, "water" type. Following are longevity tips for each constitutional body type.

Body Type: Wood.
Best Advice: Relax

Wood types (rectangular face shape) are prone to liver and gall bladder imbalances as well as cardiovascular disorders such as heart attacks, hypertension, and stroke. The personality tends to be high-strung, impatient, assertive, and competitive, predisposing wood types to nervous disorders such as mania, depression, and panic attacks. Problems with muscles, tendons, and nails may be common. Rest and relaxation are key to keeping the wood type from going up in flames. Stress release meditation and tai chi will also help counterbalance this high-strung constitution. If you recognize yourself as this type, you'd be well advised to minimize alcohol, red meat, and fatty foods.

Body Type: Metal.
Best Advice: Exercise

People who are metal types (square face shape) follow law and order. Almost engineer-like, they are precise, organized, methodical, and often idealistic. These cerebral, logical perfectionists may dwell too much in the intellect and lose touch with their feelings and physicality. Consequently, repressed or unacknowledged feelings, especially sadness and grief, can lead to stress and a weakened immune system. Metal types are prone to problems with the lungs, sinuses, throat, intestines, and skin. If you're a metal type, regular exercise will help to balance body and mind. Try using art to express feelings, and avoid overly spicy, highly processed, or refined foods.

Body Type: Fire.
Best Advice: Calm

If you're a fire type (inverted triangular face shape), you're attentive to minute details, passionate, charismatic, and spontaneous. Fire types are also very creative, their minds constantly at work. They're empathetic and connect with people on the emotional level. They are, however, prone to heart problems, especially palpitations and fast heartbeat, and tend to develop circulation problems such as varicose veins. Emotional breakdowns, anxiety, and overexcitement sometimes disrupt their lives. Fire types often have a hard time sleeping and tend to run on nervous energy. Does the shoe fit? If so, you need a stable, calm, and supportive lifestyle and will benefit from avoiding excessive excitement in your life and stimulants in your diet.

Body Type: Earth.
Best Advice: No More Sugar

The earth types (inverted trapezoid face shape) are caretakers, like the earth energy they embody. They are generally well liked, have easygoing personalities, and willingly make personal sacrifices to enable a good friend or family member to achieve a personal goal. Yet earth types tend to worry incessantly and are prone to developing digestive problems, overweight, and low energy. Bloating, water retention, and muscle aches are common. Giving freely of themselves to others, they gravitate toward food for their own fulfillment. Earth type, do your best to avoid sugar, sweets, and refined carbohydrates like breads, pasta, and pastry. Learn to say no to others' requests, to avoid depleting your energy. Remind yourself to be more spontaneous, playful, and physical.

Body Type: Water.
Best Advice: Less Salt

Those who are water types (oval face shape) are intro-
spective, mysterious, and truth seekers. They tend to be
highly imaginative, original, and possessed of a strong
sex drive. Water types like to be self-sufficient, disdain
waste, and do not give up easily. They may struggle with
loneliness and isolation, because they can be critical and
find it hard to share with others. This body type is prone
to disorders of the kidneys, bladder, and reproductive
systems and may have back pain, poor teeth, and memory
loss. Hormonal imbalance is another common issue
here. Chinese tradition advises avoiding salt in your diet
and adding more sweetness in your social life. Finally,
finding spiritual connection is key to your fulfillment.

Listen to
Your Inner Wisdom

We've all heard stories about centenarians who attribute
their longevity to a quirky practice: perhaps it's drinking a
shot of whiskey every day, walking five miles before breakfast, even saying a particular prayer. Such things are not
recommended for everyone, especially those who have not
been doing them before. But most of us have a routine or
practice that nurtures and sustains us, even if we don't
know why on an intellectual level. The action may not fit
into the framework of any dogma or philosophy; instead
it is completely personal, a ritual that is just for you. Be
attentive to your habits. Learn to distinguish between petty,
meaningless addictions and practices that help you thrive.

Word
of Mouth

There is an old Chinese saying: Most disease comes from things that enter the mouth, most trouble comes from words that leave it. The first part is easy to understand: eat wholesome, natural food and you'll have a healthy body and a clear mind. But how many people take as much care with their thoughts before they emerge as words? Most of us have experienced regret for things we have said or did not say. Be honest when you convey your feelings, be kind when you criticize something or someone, be positive when expressing your ideas, be receptive when hearing criticism, and be humble on the subject of your own virtues. By wise management of the food that enters your body and the words that leave your mouth, you will have physical vitality and peace in your heart.

Emotional Extremes Can Kill

In the Chinese healing tradition, emotions are seen to have an influence on the internal organs and vice versa. Experiencing emotions is, of course, a normal part of life, but extremes can induce imbalance and illness, including fatal disease. Excesses in the seven emotions are linked to specific organs: anger affects the liver and gall bladder; overexuberant joy (mania) can unbalance the heart and small intestine; sadness and grief disrupt the lungs and large intestine; pensiveness (overthinking, worrying) unsettles the spleen and stomach; chronic fear (insecurity) and fright (shock) both affect the kidneys and bladder. When you are visited by emotional extremes, use deep breathing and rest to restore your metabolic equilibrium. Better yet, meditate on a daily basis and head off such spikes before they start.

CHAPTER 6: Bringing It All Together:

Achieving a Fulfilling Life and Personal Legacy

To have a fulfilling life is a universal human desire. Such a life is defined by many attributes. By writing this book, I have tried to make it as easy as possible for you to achieve health, wellness, and longevity. Now it is your turn to act, to fulfill your potential by applying the knowledge you have learned. In your quest to optimize who and where you are as well as what you eat and do, the holistic approach of this book can serve as your foundation.

The most basic of attributes for a fulfilling life is health. By reading this book you can learn how to attain optimum health by decreasing disease risks through the combined wisdom of East and West. The time-tested traditions of the ancients coupled with the advancements of modern science are blended in this approach to health. Longevity is only a by-product of excellent health, which is the basis from which you can enjoy your life's true potential.

Other attributes of a fulfilling life include joy, love, freedom, prosperity, meaning, wisdom, and many more. To take joy in everyday life is a blessing that is available to all. It requires a strong desire and willingness to change in order

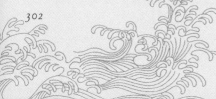

to create the joy you want. If you are unhappy, choose to be otherwise. You have that power, because no one can make you unhappy: only you determine how you feel. Commit to infusing your life and that of others with joy.

To love and be loved are crucial, because love is fundamental to all life. It starts with the benevolent love from the universal divine or God, expressed through maternal love toward children, and the goodness all human beings can feel toward one another as well as all living and nonliving things. Love's alchemy brings about the attraction between two people that inspires them to come together and form a family—the building block of the eternal universe. It is also the feeling that causes people to grow and share in community, supporting one another in life.

Freedom is something taken for granted in the developed countries of the world. The basic freedoms to think, to speak, and to be are to be valued and preserved, as they allow us all to develop as unique individuals, collectively making up the diverse world in which we live. Cultivate in your body freedom from illness, in your mind freedom from prejudice, and in your spirit freedom from the bondage of religious cults and fundamentalism—then you will taste true freedom without limit.

Another basic attribute is prosperity, and this is meant in both the material and the nonmaterial sense. Material goods are necessary for a comfortable and secure life, and it is right to be motivated to work hard in exchange for a decent living. Being creative and productive benefits you and others. We also need intangible prosperity, or good-will. Accumulating goodwill is part of human nature. Goodwill is like nutrition for the soul: the more you accrue, the more content you become.

Life without meaning is empty, but meaning is something you must give your own life. It is not for anyone else to tell you what your life is about. Take time to explore and define your life's purpose. Is your life like that of the ant scurrying about looking for food or of a butterfly dancing amid blossoms without a care? Ants and butterflies have their role to play in our planet's ecology and in the universe. The difference between humans and insects is the freedom to choose your life's mission. What is the role and purpose of your existence? When you find that mission and commit your energy to fulfilling it, your life will be fulfilled.

It has been said that everyone wants health and wisdom. Wisdom is not easily definable, yet everyone seeks it, regarding it as the highest human achievement. The funny thing is that wisdom usually does not appear until you are older, and yet no one wants to be older. Wisdom is essential to achieve health, and staying healthy in turn enables you to maximize your life span and acquire yet more wisdom. Through the continual lessons and practice of living a balanced and harmonious life, as well as cultivating your spirit, the wisdom in you grows with each passing day. And with it comes the obligation to share your wisdom in the form of service to others.

Finally we come to the subject most people would rather avoid but unfortunately is unavoidable. Let us visualize that as a result of following the advice in this book you are at the end of a long, healthy, meaningful, and productive life, and you are face to face with death. Because of the spirituality you have developed throughout your life, your soul will evolve and return to the infinite universe from whence you came, but your physical existence will cease. Will it be a quick and effortless exit or a slow and painful departure? If you have done your best to live your life in a healthy and natural way, chances are you will have a peaceful end. The cause of death will be old age and the process of dying swift.

I suggest that as a useful exercise, you start with the end in mind. Go through your life as if you are watching a movie. How would you like to be remembered? What deeds, what legacy are you leaving behind? Is the world you are departing a better place because of you? Whom do you see surrounding you at that moment? What kind of meaningful relationships did you experience in your life? In whose lives did you make a difference? Do you feel content and joyous and ready to rejoin the divine realm?

In a way, you achieve immortality through your legacy. To construct a legacy, you will need time.

May you live a long and happy life!

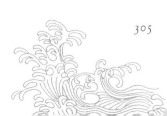

Resources

AskDrMao.com

The official Web site of *Secrets of Longevity*. Find new tips for living a long, healthy, and happy life. You can also get answers from Dr. Mao on anti-aging secrets and tools for healthy living by subscribing to his e-mail newsletters here.

www.askdrmao.com

Acupuncture.com

The oldest, most comprehensive, and most informative Web site on the Internet for acupuncture, Chinese herbal medicine, nutrition, tuina body work, tai chi, qigong, and related practices. This excellent resource for both consumers and practitioners offers access to hundreds of publications and herbal products.

www.acupuncture.com

info@acupuncture.com

Administration on Aging, Department of Health and Human Services

For more than thirty-five years, the AOA has provided home- and community-based services to millions of seniors through programs funded under the Older Americans Act. The AOA's Web site is full of useful information on various topics related to aging.

330 Independence Ave. SW, Suite 4760
Washington, DC 20201

www.aoa.gov

AoAInfo@aoa.hhs.gov

American Academy of Anti-Aging Medicine

An organization with a membership of 11,500 physicians and scientists from sixty-five countries, the American Academy of Anti-Aging Medicine (A4M) is a medical society dedicated to the advancement of therapeutics related to the science of longevity medicine. Its Web site contains a wealth of research articles related to longevity and anti-aging therapeutics. It also conducts anti-aging conferences around the world.

1510 W. Montana St.
Chicago, IL 60614

www.worldhealth.net

info@worldhealth.net

bWell

Research and treatment center for exposure to environmental toxins such a PCBs, dioxins, heavy metals, and illicit drugs. Founded by UCLA toxicologist Dr. James Dahlgreen of *Erin Brockovich* fame, the center offers a scientifically proven detoxification and wellness program that integrates Eastern and Western methods that rid the body of up to 60 percent of fat soluble chemicals and toxins.

2811 Wilshire Blvd., Suite 540
Santa Monica, CA 90403

www.bwellclinic.com
info@bwellclinic.com

Center for Food Safety

A nonprofit organization fighting for strong organic standards, promoting sustainable agriculture, and protecting consumers from the hazards of pesticides and genetically engineered food.

60 Pennsylvania Ave. SE, #302
Washington, DC 20003

www.centerforfoodsafety.org
office@centerforfoodsafety.org

Center for Mind-Body Medicine

A nonprofit educational organization founded by Dr. James Gordon and dedicated to reviving the spirit and transforming the practice of medicine. The center works to create a more effective, comprehensive, and compassionate model of health care and education, combining the precision of modern science with the best of the world's healing traditions.

5225 Connecticut Ave. NW, Suite 414
Washington, DC 20015

www.cmbm.org

The Chopra Center

Retreat and spa founded by Dr. Deepak Chopra located in San Diego, California. It offers a wide range of health and rejuvenation services based on integrating allopathic and Indian ayurvedic traditions.

2013 Costa del Mar Rd.
Carlsbad, CA 92009

www.chopra.com
info@chopra.com

Environmental Protection Agency

The EPA's mission is to protect human health and the environment. Since 1970, the agency has been working for a cleaner, healthier environment in the United States. The EPA leads the nation's environmental science, research, education, and assessment efforts. You can find useful information about radon and other environmental pollutants here.

Ariel Rios Building
1200 Pennsylvania Ave. NW
Washington, DC 20460

www.epa.gov

Gerontology Research Group

A group of professors, research scientists, and doctors sharing the latest findings as well as thought-provoking opinions on aging and life-extension techniques. Founded by Dr. L. Stephen Coles, MD, PhD, a professor and researcher in stem cell technology and longevity medicine at the University of California at Los Angeles School of Medicine, it also hosts monthly forums open to the public on the UCLA campus.

P.O. Box 905
Santa Clarita, CA 91380-9005

www.grg.org

The Grain and Salt Society

Offers unrefined sea salts, organic bulk whole foods, traditional cookware, hygiene products and books.

4 Celtic Dr.
Arden, NC 28704

www.celtic-seasalt.com
info@celtic-seasalt.com

Healing People Network

Comprehensive Web site on complementary and alternative medicine (CAM) for consumers and practitioners. In-depth coverage of subjects such as acupuncture, aromatherapy, ayurveda, bodywork, Chinese medicine, cancer risk reduction, environmental toxicology, fitness training, herbalism, homeopathy, naturopathy, nutrition and lifestyle, pet health, and other natural healing modalities. The site also provides a referral network of CAM practitioners throughout the United States and access to more than 1,000 pharmaceutical-grade supplement products.

906 E. Verdugo Rd.
Burbank, CA 91501

www.healingpeople.com
contact@healingpeople.com

Herb Research Foundation

Provides useful information on well-researched therapeutic herbs and publishes an herb magazine, *HerbalGram*.

4140 15th St.
Boulder, CO 80304

www.herbs.org

National Council on Aging

Founded in 1950, the National Council on Aging is a national network of organizations and individuals dedicated to improving the health and independence of older persons and increasing their continuing contributions to communities, society, and future generations.

300 D Street SW, Suite 801
Washington, DC 20024

www.ncoa.gov

info@ncoa.gov

Natural Resource Defense Council

NRDC is one of the nation's most effective environmental action organizations. It employs law, science, and the support of more than a million members and online activists to protect the planet's wildlife and wild places and to ensure a safe, healthy environment for all living things. The council also publishes a useful monthly newsletter.

40 W. 20th St.
New York, NY 10011

www.nrdc.org
nrdcinfo@nrdc.org

Tao of Wellness

Health and wellness centers in Southern California that specialize in providing quality service in acupuncture and Chinese medicine. Co-founded by Dr. Maoshing Ni.

1131 Wilshire Blvd., Suite 300
Santa Monica, CA 90401

www.taoofwellness.com
contact@taoofwellness.com

U.S. Consumer Products Safety Commission

The CPSC's primary goals are to protect the public against unreasonable risks of injuries associated with consumer products, develop uniform safety standards, and promote research and investigation into the prevention of product-related death, injury, and illness. The commission puts out free fact sheets on hazardous products.

Washington, DC 20207

www.cpsc.gov

Weil Lifestyle LLC

The organization of Andrew Weil, MD, publishes the popular *Self Healing* newsletter and maintains a Web site that is the leading online resource for healthy living based on integrative medicine. Also provides e-mailed daily tips and weekly health updates.

www.drweil.com

contact@drweil.com

Whole Foods Market

Founded in 1980 as one small store in Austin, Texas, Whole Foods Market is now the world's leading retailer of natural and organic foods, with more than 170 stores in North America and the United Kingdom. These stores are a good place for healthy, mostly organic food, dietary supplements, and household cleaning supplies.

525 N. Lamar
Austin, TX 78703

www.wholefoods.com

Wild Oats Market

Founded in 1987 as Crystal Market, this was the only vegetarian natural food store in Boulder, Colorado. Wild Oats is now the second largest retailer of natural and organic foods, with more than 100 stores in North America. Healthy natural and organic food, supplements, and household supplies.

3375 Mitchell Lane
Boulder, CO 80301

www.wildoats.com

World Research Foundation

WRF established a unique, international health information network to help people stay informed of all available treatments around the world. The nonprofit is one of the only groups that provides health information on both allopathic and alternative medicine techniques.

41 Bell Rock Plaza
Sedona, AZ 86351

www.wrf.org

info@wrf.org

Yo San University

An accredited graduate school of traditional Chinese medicine founded by Dr. Maoshing Ni and his family. Its rigorous academic, clinical, and spiritual development programs train students for the professional practice of acupuncture and Eastern medicine. Its ongoing community-based Healthy Aging Initiative is funded by a research grant from the Unihealth Foundation.

13315 W. Washington Blvd., Suite 200
Los Angeles, CA 90066

www.yosan.edu

admissions@yosan.edu

Bibliography

Adlercreutz, Herman. "Lignans and Phytoestrogens: Possible Protective Role in Cancer." *Frontiers of Gastrointestinal Research*, 1988, 14:165–176.

Anderson, James W. "Dietary Fiber and Diabetes." *Journal of the American Dietetic Association*, September 1987, 9:1189–1197.

Anderson, R. A., et al. "Chromium Supplementation of Human Subjects: Effects on Glucose, Insulin, and Lipid Variables." *Metabolism*, 1983, 32:894–899.

Anti-Aging Therapeutics. Volumes 2–6. Chicago, IL: A4M Publications. 1999–2004. CD-ROM.

Baker, Sidney MacDonald, with Karen Baar. *The Circadian Prescription*. New York: Perigee Books, 2000.

Balch, James F., and Phyllis A. Balch. *Prescription for Nutritional Healing*. New York: Avery Publishing Group, 1990.

Barbul, Adrian, et al. "Arginine Stimulates Lymphocyte Immune Response in Healthy Human Beings." *Surgery*, 1981, 90: 244–251.

"Be Your Best: Nutrition After Fifty." Washington, DC: American Institute for Cancer Research, 1988.

Borek, Carmia. *Maximize Your Health-Span with Antioxidants*. New Canaan, CT: Keats Publishing, 1995.

Bowman, Barbara. "Acetyl-Carnitine and Alzheimer's Disease." *Nutrition Review*, 1992, 50:142–144.

Brody, Jane. "Restoring Ebbing Hormones May Slow Aging." *New York Times*, July 18, 1995.

Caragay, Alegria B. "Cancer-Preventive Foods and Ingredients." *Food Technology*, April 1992, 46: 65–68.

Cerda, J. J., et al. "The Effects of Grapefruit Pectin on Patients at Risk for Coronary Heart Disease without Altering Diet or Lifestyle." *Clinical Cardiology*, September 1988, 9:589–594.

Chen, K. J., and K. Chen. "Ischemic Stroke Treated with Ligusticum Chuanxiong." *Chinese Medical Journal*, October 1992, 10:870–873.

Chopra, Deepak. *Ageless Body, Timeless Mind: The Quantum Alternative to Growing Old*. New York: Harmony, 1994.

——. *The Book of Secrets: Unlocking the Hidden Dimensions of Your Life*. New York: Harmony, 2004.

——. *Grow Younger, Live Longer: Ten Steps to Reverse Aging*. New York: Three Rivers Press, 2002.

"Chronic Stress Is Directly Linked to Premature Aging of the Brain." National Institute on Aging Research Bulletin, October 1991.

Cole, Stephen. "CoQ-10 and Life Span Extension." *Journal of Longevity Research*, 1995, 1(5):221–223.

Cryer, Sibyl. "New Music and Stress Reduction Technique Increase Anti-aging Hormone—DHEA." Institute of Heartmath, July 19, 1995, 1–2.

Cutler, Richard G. "Antioxidants and Aging." *American Journal of Clinical Nutrition*, 1991, 53:373S–379S.

Dadd, Debra Lynn. *The Non-Toxic Home: Protecting Yourself and Your Family from Everyday Toxins and Health Hazards.* Los Angeles: Jeremy P. Tarcher, Inc., 1986.

"Diet and Cancer." American Institute for Cancer Research Information Series, 1992.

"Diet, Nutrition, and Prostate Cancer." American Institute for Cancer Research Information Series, 1991.

Dilman, V., et al. "The Neuroendocrine Theory of Aging and Degenerative Disease." Pensacola, FL: Center for Bio-Gerontology, 1992.

Duke, James A. "An Herb a Day: Clubmoss, Alias Lycopodium Alias Huperzia." *Business of Herbs*, January/February 1989, 5–8.

——.*The Green Pharmacy Anti-Aging Prescriptions: Herbs, Foods, and Natural Formulas to Keep You Young.* Emmaus, PA: Rodale Books, 2001.

Evans, W. J. "Exercise, Nutrition and Aging." Symposium: Nutrition and Exercise, *Journal of Nutrition*, 1992, 122:796–801.

Evergreen Secrets: You Can Live to 120. Taipei, Taiwan: Taiwan TV Media Company, 1989.

Farlow, Christine. *Dying to Look Good: The Disturbing Truth About What's Really in Your Cosmetics, Toiletries and Personal Care Products.* Escondido, CA: KISS for Health Publishing, 2001.

Feldman, Henry A., et al. "Impotence and Its Medical and Psychosocial Correlates: Results of the Massachusetts Male Aging Study." *Journal of Urology*, January 1994, 151:54–61.

Fiatarone, Maria, Evelyn F. O'Neill, and Nancy Doyle Ryan. "Exercise Training and Nutritional Supplementation for Physical Frailty in Very Elderly People." *New England Journal of Medicine*, June 23, 1994, 25:1769–1775.

Ford, Norman. *Lifestyle for Longevity.* Gloucester, MA: Para Research, 1984.

Gaby, Alan R. "DHEA: The Hormone That Does It All." *Holistic Medicine*, Spring 1993, 19–22.

"Garlic, Tomatoes and Other Produce Fight Nitrosamine Formation." *Science News*, 1991, 145:190.

"Ginger and Atractylodes as an Anti-inflammatory." *HerbalGram*, 1993, 29:19.

Gordon, James S. *Comprehensive Cancer Care: Integrating Alternative, Complementary and Conventional Therapy.* New York: Perseus Books Group, 2000.

———. *Manifesto for a New Medicine: Your Guide to Healing Partnerships and the Wise Use of Alternative Therapies.* Boston: Addison Wesley Publishing Company, 1997.

Graf, Ernst, and John W. Eaton. "Antioxidant Functions of Phytic Acid." *Free Radical Biology and Medicine,* 1990, 8:61–69.

Haas, Elson M. *Staying Healthy with Nutrition.* Berkeley, CA: Celestial Arts, 1992.

———. *Staying Healthy with the Seasons.* Berkeley, CA: Celestial Arts, 1981.

Hayflick, L. *How and Why We Age.* New York: Ballantine Books, 1994.

"Herbs and Spices May Be Barrier Against Cancer, Heart Disease." *Environmental Nutrition,* June 1993, 54–57.

Hobbs, Christopher, and Steven Foster. "Hawthorn: A Literature Review." *HerbalGram,* Spring 1990, 22:19–33.

Inlander, Charles B., and Marie Hodge. *100 Ways to Live to 100: How to Live a Century.* Allentown, PA: People's Medical Society, 1992.

Jain, Adesh K., et al. "Can Garlic Reduce Levels of Serum Lipids? A Controlled Clinical Study." *American Journal of Medicine,* June 1993, 94:632–635.

Jenson, Bernard Anderson, and Mark Anderson. *Empty Harvest: Understanding the Link Between Our Food, Our Immunity, and Our Planet.* New York: Avery Publishing Group, 1990.

Johnston, Carol S., Claudia Meyer, and J. C. Srilakshmi. "Vitamin C Elevates Red Blood Cell Glutathione in Healthy Adults." *American Journal of Clinical Nutrition,* 1993, 58:103–105.

Kamikawa, Todashi, et al. "Effects of Coenzyme Q10 on Exercise Tolerance in Chronic Stable Angina Pectoris." *American Journal of Cardiology,* 1985, 56:247–251.

Kaufman, Richard C. *The Age Reduction System.* New York: Rawson Associates, 1986.

Keough, Carol. *The Complete Book of Cancer Prevention.* Emmaus, PA: Rodale Press, 1988.

Khan, A., et al. "Insulin Potentiating Factor and Chromium Content of Selected Foods and Spices." *Biologic Trace Element Research,* March 1990, 3:183–188.

Klatz, Ronald M., and Robert Goldman. *Stopping the Clock.* New Canaan, CT: Keats Publishing, 1996.

Klatz, Ronald M., et al. "Cellular Phone Radiation and Potential Risks to the Human Brain: A Review of Scientific Literature." *Anti-Aging Medical News,* Winter 2002, 1–12.

Kotulak, Ronald, and Peter Gorner. *Aging on Hold.* New York: Tribune Publishing, 1992.

Kronhausen, E., P. Kronhausen, and H. Demopoulos. *Formulas for Life.* New York: William Morrow, 1989.

Lipkin, Richard. "Wine's Chemical Secrets." *Science News,* October 23, 1993, 144: 264–265.

McCaleb, Rob. "Astragalus." *Herb Information Green Paper*, Herb Research Foundation. May 5, 2003.

McGraw, Phillip C. *Self Matters: Creating Your Life from the Inside Out*. New York: Free Press, 2003.

Merimee, T. J., et al. "Arginine-Initiated Release of Growth Hormone: Factors Modifying the Response in Normal Men." *New England Journal of Medicine*, 1969, 280(26): 1434–1438.

Mindell, Earl. *Earl Mindell's Anti-Aging Bible*. New York: Fireside, 1996.

"Mining for Toxic Minerals Hidden in Our Diets." *Environmental Nutrition*, March 1992, 15(3): 32–34.

Nelson, M., E. Fisher, F. Dilmanian, G. Dallal, and W. Evans. "A 1-Year Walking Program and Increased Dietary Calcium in Postmenopausal Women: Effects on Bone." *American Journal of Clinical Nutrition*, 1991, 53:1304–1311.

Ni, Hua-Ching. *The Complete Works of Lao Tzu: Tao Teh Ching and Hua Hu Ching*. Los Angeles: Seven Star Communications, 2000.

——. *Enrich Your Life with Virtue*. Los Angeles: Seven Star Communications, 1999.

——. *Foundation of a Happy Life*. Los Angeles: Seven Star Communications, 1999.

——. *Harmony: The Art of Life*. Los Angeles: Shrine of Eternal Breath of Tao/College of Tao and Traditional Chinese Healing, 1991.

——. *Power of Natural Healing*. Los Angeles: Seven Star Communications, 1990.

——. *Tao: The Subtle Universal Law and the Integral Way of Life*. Los Angeles: Seven Star Communications, 1998.

——. *Workbook for Spiritual Development*. Los Angeles: Seven Star Communications, 1995.

Ni, Hua-Ching, with Daoshing Ni and Maoshing Ni. *Strength from Movement: Mastering Chi*. Los Angeles: Seven Star Communications, 1990.

Ni, Hua-Ching, and Maoshing Ni. *The Power of the Feminine*. Los Angeles: Seven Star Communications, 1990.

Ni, Maoshing. *Chinese Herbology Made Easy*. Los Angeles: Seven Star Communications, 2003.

——. *The Yellow Emperor's Classic of Medicine: A New Translation of the Neijing Suwen with Commentary*. Boston: Shambhala, 1995.

Ni, Maoshing, and Cathy McNease. *The Tao of Nutrition*. Los Angeles: Seven Star Communications, 1993.

Oschman, James L. *Energy Medicine: The Scientific Basis*. New York: Churchill Livingstone, 2000.

Pitchford, Paul. *Healing with Whole Foods*. Berkeley, CA: North Atlantic Books, 2002.

Reid, Daniel. *The Tao of Health, Sex and Longevity*. New York: Fireside Books, 1989.

Rothenberg, Ron, and Kathleen Becker. "Forever Ageless." Encinitas, CA: HealthSpan Institute, 2001.

Rudman, D., et al. "Effects of Human Growth Hormone in Men over 60 Years Old." *New England Journal of Medicine*, 1990, 323:1–6.

Rusting, Ricki L. "Why Do We Age?" *Scientific American*, December 1992, 267(1):131–141.

Sears, Barry. *The Anti-Aging Zone*. New York: Regan Books, 1998.

Selkoe, Dennis J. "Aging Brain, Aging Mind: Structural and Chemical Changes." *Scientific American*, September 1992, 267(3): 134–142.

Shepard, Roy J. "Exercise and Aging: Extending independence in Older Adults." *Geriatrics*, May 1993, 48(5):61–64.

Simopoulos, Artemis P. "Omega-3 Fatty Acids in Health and Disease and in Growth and Development." *American Journal of Clinical Nutrition*, 1991, 54:438–463.

Smith, Timothy J. *Renewal: The Anti-Aging Revolution*. New York: St. Martin's Press, 1999.

Smolensky, Michael, and Lynne Lamberg. *The Body Clock Guide to Better Health*. New York: Henry Holt and Company, 2000.

Stern, Yaakov, et al. "Influence of Education and Occupation on the Incidence of Alzheimer's Disease." *Journal of the American Medical Association*, April 6, 1994, 1,004–10.

Sun, Jian Ming, et al. *Secrets of Longevity throughout Chinese History*. Xian, China: Tienze Publisher, 1989.

Tkac, Debora, ed. *Life Span Plus*. New York: MJF Books, 1990.

Travis, John W., and Regina Sara Ryan. *Wellness Workbook: How to Achieve Enduring Health and Vitality*. Berkeley, CA: Celestial Arts, 2004.

Tucker, Don M., et al. "Nutrition Status and Brain Function in Aging." *American Journal of Clinical Nutrition*, 1990, 52:93–102.

"23-Year Study of Middle-Aged Men in Hawaii Confirms: Physical Activity Will Lower Risk of Heart Disease." *News from the American Heart Association*, June 13, 1994, 2,540–44.

Ullis, Karlis. *Age Right: Turn Back the Clock with a Proven, Personalized, Anti-Aging Program*. New York: Simon & Schuster, 1999.

U.S. Department of Agriculture. "Nutritive Value of American Foods in Common Units." Agriculture Handbook No. 456, 1975.

Walford, Roy L., and Lisa Walford. *The Anti-Aging Plan: The Nutrient-Rich, Low-Calorie Way of Eating for a Longer Life—The Only Diet Scientifically Proven to Extend Your Healthy Years*. New York: Marlowe & Company, 2005.

Warner, H. R., R. N. Butler, R. C. Sprott, and E. L. Schneider. *Modern Biological Theories of Aging*. New York: Raven Press, 1987.

Wei-Hua, Lu, Jiang Shou, and Xi-Can Tang. "Improving Effect of Huperzine A on Discrimination Performance in Aged Rats and Adult Rats with Experimental Cognitive Impairment." *Acta Pharmacologica Sinica*, January 1988, 1:11–15.

Weil, Andrew T. *Eating Well For Optimum Health: The Essential Guide to Bringing Health and Pleasure Back to Eating*. New York: Perennial Currents, 2001.

———. *8 Weeks to Optimum Health*. New York: Ballantine Books, 1998.

———. *Natural Health, Natural Medicine: The Complete Guide to Wellness and Self-Care for Optimum Health*. New York: Houghton Mifflin, 2004.

———. *Perfect Health: The Complete Mind/Body Guide*. New York: Harmony, 2001.

Whitaker, Julian. *Reversing Heart Disease*. New York: Warner Books, 1985.

Wild, Russell, ed., et al. *The Complete Book of Natural and Medicinal Cures*. Emmaus, PA: Rodale Press, 1994.

Williams, Gurney. "Mind, Body, Spirit: Portable Meditation, Stress Relief for Those on the Go." *Longevity*, May 1993, p. 72.

Yao, Congli, and Ming Liu. *Health Preservation and Longevity*. Beijing, China: Popular Science Press, 1985. (In Chinese)

Yeager, Selene, et al. *New Foods for Healing*. Emmaus, PA: Rodale Press, 1998.

Zhang, Rongcai, ed. *Eldercare and Longevity*. Fujian, China: Fujian Science and Technology Press, 1987. (In Chinese)

Index

325

Acknowledgments

*There are many people who have been instrumental in the
ultimate publication of this book. First of all, without the
incredible support and understanding from my wife, Emm,
and our children, Yu-Shien Michelle, Yu-Shing Natasha, and
Yu-Kai Nicholas, during the period of writing this book, in
which they endured my absence from our routine interactions,
I would not have undertaken this project. I am lucky and
grateful that they are in my life.*

*The data on centenarians I collected over the last twenty years
would still be sitting in my study if it weren't for the persistent
efforts of Stuart Shapiro, who brought Laurie Dolphin and
myself together; the relationship that made this book take
shape. I am thankful to both for their unwavering belief in me.*

*I am deeply appreciative to Laurie Dolphin, my collaborator
who has been my cheerleader the whole way, helping to coor-
dinate every aspect of the book from the beginning to the end
and whose professional talents are displayed throughout the
book in its tasteful design and layout.*

*I am indebted to Jodi Davis, our editor at Chronicle Books,
who suggested the format and guided our vision for the even-
tual book. I am thankful for her patience for putting up with
my busy schedule and sheparding the project through its
many twists and turns.*

*A special thanks goes to Elizabeth Bell, our copyeditor, who
went beyond more than what is normally required of her job
and painstakingly rewrote many of the tips to make the book*

flow better. Also thanks to Allison Meierding, Laurie's assistant, whose tireless dedication in the project helped it to come to fruition.

I have Dr. Andrew Weil, Dr. Deepak Chopra, and Dr. James Gordon to thank for their pioneering work that brought the movement of natural medicine to the forefront of mainstream awareness. Their individual and collective voices have helped usher in the integration of Eastern and Western health traditions and the creation of a new health and wellness paradigm in the West.

I owe many thanks to the centenarians and patients who generously shared with me their stories and personal longevity secrets. I am also indebted to the long and rich tradition of Chinese Taoists, represented by masters such as the Yellow Emperor, Lao Tzu, and Ge Hong, whose 8,000-year quests for immortality left behind many longevity secrets, many of which found their way into this book.

Finally, I thank the divine universal origin and my parents for the genesis of my life and for their determined efforts to restore me from my near-death experience as a child. Their nurturing and teaching inspired me to seek the knowledge and wisdom of health, wellness, and longevity for the benefit of the whole world.

Dedication

This book is dedicated to those who seek to live well,
live long, and live happily.